GW00993220

Influence (Pregnancy Weiym on Maternal and Child Health

WORKSHOP REPORT

Committee on the Impact of Pregnancy Weight
on Maternal and Child Health

Board on Children, Youth, and Families
Division of Behavioral and Social Sciences and Education
Institute of Medicine

Food and Nutrition Board
Institute of Medicine

NATIONAL RESEARCH COUNCIL
INSTITUTE OF MEDICINE
OF THE NATIONAL ACADEMIES

THE NATIONAL ACADEMIES PRESS
Washington, D.C.
www.nap.edu

THE NATIONAL ACADEMIES PRESS   500 Fifth Street, N.W.   Washington, DC 20001

NOTICE: The project that is the subject of this report was approved by the Governing Board of the National Research Council, whose members are drawn from the councils of the National Academy of Sciences, the National Academy of Engineering, and the Institute of Medicine. The members of the committee responsible for the report were chosen for their special competences and with regard for appropriate balance.

This study was supported by Award No. HHSH24055014 between the National Academy of Sciences and the Department of Health and Human Services. Any opinions, findings, conclusions, or recommendations expressed in this publication are those of the author(s) and do not necessarily reflect the views of the organizations or agencies that provided support for the project.

International Standard Book Number 13: 978-0-309-10406-7
International Standard Book Number 10: 0-309-10406-8

Additional copies of this report are available from the National Academies Press, 500 Fifth Street, N.W., Lockbox 285, Washington, DC 20055; (800) 624-6242 or (202) 334-3313 (in the Washington metropolitan area); Internet, http://www.nap.edu

Printed in the United States of America

Suggested citation: National Research Council and Institute of Medicine. (2007). *Influence of Pregnancy Weight on Maternal and Child Health. Workshop Report.* Committee on the Impact of Pregnancy Weight on Maternal and Child Health. Board on Children, Youth, and Families, Division of Behavioral and Social Sciences and Education and Food and Nutrition Board, Institute of Medicine. Washington, DC: The National Academies Press.

THE NATIONAL ACADEMIES
Advisers to the Nation on Science, Engineering, and Medicine

The **National Academy of Sciences** is a private, nonprofit, self-perpetuating society of distinguished scholars engaged in scientific and engineering research, dedicated to the furtherance of science and technology and to their use for the general welfare. Upon the authority of the charter granted to it by the Congress in 1863, the Academy has a mandate that requires it to advise the federal government on scientific and technical matters. Dr. Ralph J. Cicerone is president of the National Academy of Sciences.

The **National Academy of Engineering** was established in 1964, under the charter of the National Academy of Sciences, as a parallel organization of outstanding engineers. It is autonomous in its administration and in the selection of its members, sharing with the National Academy of Sciences the responsibility for advising the federal government. The National Academy of Engineering also sponsors engineering programs aimed at meeting national needs, encourages education and research, and recognizes the superior achievements of engineers. Dr. Wm. A. Wulf is president of the National Academy of Engineering.

The **Institute of Medicine** was established in 1970 by the National Academy of Sciences to secure the services of eminent members of appropriate professions in the examination of policy matters pertaining to the health of the public. The Institute acts under the responsibility given to the National Academy of Sciences by its congressional charter to be an adviser to the federal government and, upon its own initiative, to identify issues of medical care, research, and education. Dr. Harvey V. Fineberg is president of the Institute of Medicine.

The **National Research Council** was organized by the National Academy of Sciences in 1916 to associate the broad community of science and technology with the Academy's purposes of furthering knowledge and advising the federal government. Functioning in accordance with general policies determined by the Academy, the Council has become the principal operating agency of both the National Academy of Sciences and the National Academy of Engineering in providing services to the government, the public, and the scientific and engineering communities. The Council is administered jointly by both Academies and the Institute of Medicine. Dr. Ralph J. Cicerone and Dr. Wm. A. Wulf are chair and vice chair, respectively, of the National Research Council.

www.national-academies.org

FOOD AND NUTRITION BOARD

Preface

This volume summarizes a one and a half day workshop convened in May 2006 that reviewed U.S. trends in maternal weight (prior to, during, and after pregnancy) among different populations of women; examined the emerging research findings related to the complex relationship of the biological, behavioral, psychological, and social interactions that affect maternal and pregnancy weight on maternal and child health outcomes; and discussed interventions that use this complex relationship to promote appropriate weight during pregnancy and postpartum.

Given the unprecedented environment in the United States in which two-thirds of the adult population meet the criteria for being overweight or obese, the implications for women in the reproductive age period are unique in the history of the country. The concerns for maternal and infant health are real. The questions and answers tackled by committee members and workshop participants were not easy. Nevertheless, having an opportunity to explore what is known, examine the gaps in knowledge, and explore what to do now and in the future builds a pathway for further inquiry and action. This report summarizes the workshop proceedings and highlights key themes that deserve further attention.

The overarching goal of the workshop was for participants to describe what is known about recent trends in maternal weight gain and the impact of maternal weight during pregnancy on the health of mothers and their children. The workshop provided a valuable opportunity to assess trends that have occurred since the publication of an earlier study by the Institute of Medicine (IOM), which included guidelines for recommended weight gain during pregnancy.[1] This report seeks to inform the efforts of Title V maternal and child health programs to foster adherence to the IOM recommendations for recommended weight gain during pregnancy as well as contribute to understanding whether there is a substantial need to reexamine these recommendations in light of recent demographic and health trends.

The genesis of the workshop began with a proposal that was reviewed and refined by the National Research Council-IOM Board on Children, Youth, and Families and the IOM Food and Nutrition Board. The Maternal and Child Health Bureau of the U.S. Department of Health and Human Services subsequently funded an activity that included the formation of a program committee that met once to help plan and convene the workshop. The efforts of the planning committee members and the workshop participants fostered a collaboration that began the unraveling of a challenging and multifaceted area of study.

We are particularly grateful for the contributions of the expert presenters, speakers, and discussants who contributed to the meeting (see the Appendix for the workshop agenda and list of participants). Special appreciation also goes to the members of the planning committee, who volunteered their time and intellectual efforts to shape the workshop program and identify themes and contributors. In addition, we give special thanks to Margaret Feerick, who prepared a comprehensive draft of the workshop report; Leslie Sim, who directed the planning and workshop preparation and the production of the final publication; and Wendy Keenan, who assisted with preparation of the workshop and the final report. Although the workshop report was prepared by the committee, it does not represent findings or recommendations that can be attributed to the committee members.

This workshop report has been reviewed in draft form by individuals chosen for their diverse perspectives and technical expertise, in accordance with procedures approved by the Report Review Committee of the National Research Council. The purpose of this independent review is to provide candid and critical comments that will assist the institution in making its published report as sound as possible and to ensure that the report meets institutional standards for objectivity, evidence, and responsiveness to the charge. The review comments and draft manuscript remain confidential to protect the integrity of the process. We thank the following individuals for their review of this report: Esa M. Davis, Department of Family Medicine-Research Division, Case Western Reserve University/ University Hospital of Cleveland; Calvin J. Hobel, Department of Obstet-

---

[1]Institute of Medicine (1990), *Nutrition During Pregnancy*. Washington, DC: National Academy Press.

rics and Gynecology, Cedars Sinai Medical Center, Los Angeles, CA; Christine M. Olson, Division of Nutritional Sciences, Cornell University; Magda G. Peck, Department of Pediatrics, University of Nebraska Medical Center; Kathryn Peppe, Program and Policy Office, Association of Maternal and Child Health Programs, Washington, DC; Nicolas Stettler, Department of Pediatrics and Epidemiology, The Children's Hospital of Philadelphia; and Brian Wrotniak, Department of Pediatrics and Epidemiology, The Children's Hospital of Philadelphia.

Although the reviewers listed above provided many constructive comments and suggestions, they were not asked to endorse the content of the report nor did they see the final draft of the report before its release. The review of this report was overseen by Thomas DeWitt, Division of General and Community Pediatrics, Cincinnati Children's Hospital Medical Center. Appointed by the National Research Council, he was responsible for making certain that an independent examination of this report was carried out in accordance with institutional procedures and that all review comments were carefully considered. Responsibility for the final content of this report rests entirely with the authors and the institution.

Maxine Hayes, *Chair*
Committee on the Impact of
  Pregnancy Weight on Maternal
  and Child Health

Contents

1

Introduction

There is a growing epidemic of obesity in the United States: nearly one-third of all adults are classified as obese, and this proportion has dramatically increased during the last two decades (Flegal et al., 2002; Hedley et al., 2004).[1] Women are leading the epidemic at a current prevalence rate of obesity of 33 percent (National Center for Health Statistics, 2004; Ogden et al., 2006).

Given the environment of overweight and obesity in the United States, the implications of this epidemic for women of childbearing age are of a concern. Data from the March of Dimes Perinatal Data Center indicate that in 2003, 19.6 percent of U.S. women of reproductive age were obese (March of Dimes, 2004). Obesity in women can cause serious pregnancy-related complications, but women can also modify their weight.

Past efforts to advise women on weight for pregnancy (before, during, and after) have focused little on maternal obesity. Rather, most of the attention has been devoted to concerns about low birth weight deliveries in addition to other maternal and infant outcomes. *Maternal Nutrition and the Course of Pregnancy*, a 1970 report of the Food and Nutrition Board of the National Research Council (NRC)[2] (National Research Council, 1970),

---

[1]Obesity is defined as having a body mass index of 30 or greater. Body mass index is a measure that appears throughout this report as the ratio of weight to height squared (kg/m^2 or $lb/in^2 \times 703$) (National Heart, Lung, and Blood Institute, 1998).

[2]The Food and Nutrition Board was once a part of the National Research Council. It is now housed in the Institute of Medicine.

laid the foundation for work over the next two decades, and in 1974, the U.S. Department of Agriculture established the Special Supplemental Food Program for Women, Infants, and Children to address the needs of women and children at nutritional risk.

In 1990 the Institute of Medicine (IOM) report *Nutrition During Pregnancy* recommended guidelines for weight gain during pregnancy based on prepregnancy maternal body mass index (BMI). Two other reports quickly followed: *Nutrition During Lactation* (1991) and *Nutrition During Pregnancy and Lactation: An Implementation Guide* (1992).

By this time, the Maternal and Child Health Bureau of the U.S. Department of Health and Human Services had also begun to address concerns about maternal weight gain. And in 1998, the National Heart, Lung, and Blood Institute (NHLBI) released its own classification of overweight and obesity by BMI (National Heart, Lung, and Blood Institute, 1998). The NHLBI classifications differed slightly from the 1990 IOM maternal BMI criteria. However, a common stimulus for all of these earlier efforts was the incidence of low birth weight deliveries, which was in part attributed to insufficient nutrition and insufficient weight gain during pregnancy.

Since publication of the 1990 IOM recommendations for weight gain during pregnancy, tremendous changes have occurred in the demographic and epidemiological profile of women experiencing pregnancy. More women entering pregnancy are either overweight or obese, and more women are entering their pregnancies with chronic conditions that lead to increased morbidity during their postpregnancy years. High rates of overweight and obesity are especially common in minority populations that may be already at risk for poor maternal and child health outcomes. Collectively, these trends have prompted concern about the adequacy of existing guidelines for weight gain during pregnancy, particularly for women who are overweight, underweight, short in stature, or adolescents.

Despite the availability of the IOM recommendations and an effort to publicize their availability, their use and compliance are not understood. As researchers have begun to address some of the issues raised in the 1990 IOM report, gaps in knowledge have emerged, even as additional data are collected and reported.

This convergence of factors prompted the NRC and the IOM to organize a workshop on maternal weight gain (before, during, and after pregnancy) and its influence on maternal and child health. With support from the Maternal and Child Health Bureau in the U.S. Department of Health and Human Services, the NRC-IOM Board on Children, Youth, and Families, in collaboration with the IOM Food and Nutrition Board, convened a committee of experts at a day and a half workshop in May 2006 to examine the current state of knowledge and highlight key observations that could form the basis for future study and deliberations regarding maternal weight gain during pregnancy (see the Appendix for the full workshop agenda and list of participants). The workshop sought to address five questions:

1.   What research and databases describe the distribution of maternal weight (prior to, during, and after pregnancy) among different populations of women in the United States?
2.   What research and databases inform understanding of the effects of different weight patterns (including underweight and overweight) during pregnancy on maternal and child health outcomes (up to 12 months)?
3.   What research has been conducted to describe the individual, community, and health care system factors that impede or foster compliance with recommended gestational weight guidelines (prior to, during, and after pregnancy)?
4.   What opportunities exist for Title V maternal and child health programs to build on this knowledge to help childbearing women achieve and maintain recommended weight (prior to, during, and after pregnancy)?
5.   What future research and data collection efforts could improve the efforts of Title V programs to support women from different racial and ethnic backgrounds in their efforts to comply with recommended weight guidelines and to improve their maternal health?

Throughout the workshop, the term "maternal weight gain" was used to refer to weight gain during different time periods of a woman's life (Box 1-1). It must be noted that in longitudinal studies and studies of women with multiple pregnancies, various terms may be used interchangeably in reference to a specific pregnancy. A woman whose second preg-

---

BOX 1-1

Maternal Weight Definitions

Prepregnancy Weight: A woman's actual weight prior to pregnancy up to the point that pregnancy is identified.

Prepregnancy Weight Gain: A woman's increase in weight from some prior time until pregnancy.

Gestational Weight Gain: Amount of weight gained during the pregnancy.

Postpartum Weight Retention: Amount of weight gained during pregnancy (i.e., gestational weight gain) that the woman has at a given time point postpartum.

Postpartum Weight Gain: Weight that is gained following pregnancy.

nancy is the focus of study, then, may have weight gained between the two pregnancies described as weight retention (from the first pregnancy), postpartum weight gain (which would also be prepregnancy weight gain in reference to the second pregnancy), and then gestational weight gain and weight retention connected with the second pregnancy.

This report documents the information presented in the workshop presentations and deliberations. Its purpose is to lay out the key ideas that emerged from the workshop, both for researchers interested in interdisciplinary work in this area and for those who are involved in developing strategies to promote appropriate weight before, during, and after pregnancy. The report should be viewed as only a first step in exploring opportunities to develop a synthesis of diverse research and applying this knowledge to promote appropriate weight in women of childbearing age, and it is confined to the material presented by the workshop speakers and participants. Neither the workshop nor this report is intended as a comprehensive review of what is known about maternal weight and gestational weight gain and maternal and child health outcomes, although it is a general reflection of the literature. Many additional contributors of gestational weight gain and health outcomes—such as food frequency, congenital malformations, gender of the infant, metabolic syndrome, and contraception—were not addressed in the limited time available for the workshop. A more comprehensive review and synthesis of relevant research knowledge will have to wait for further development. Although this report was prepared by the committee, it does not represent findings or recommendations that can be attributed to the committee members. Indeed, the report summarized views expressed by workshop participants and the committee is responsible only for its overall quality and accuracy as a record of what transpired at the workshop. The workshop was not designed to generate consensus conclusions or recommendations but focused instead on the identification of ideas, themes, and considerations that contribute to understanding the role of weight gain during pregnancy as well as informing strategies that might help women achieve and maintain appropriate weight. The workshop mainly considered health outcomes of public health significance for the United States and is not necessarily pertinent to other settings.

One additional topic deserves attention in presenting this overview of pregnancy weight gain studies. Various presenters referred to weight patterns measured in pounds or kilograms. In this report, all data are reported in pound measures. Data that refer to kilogram measures have been converted to pounds to allow for easier comparisons across research studies.

Following this introduction, the report includes five sections that highlight the panel presentations at the workshop: (1) trends in maternal and gestational weight, (2) determinants of gestational weight gain, (3) consequences of gestational weight gain for maternal health, (4) infant health outcomes that ensue from maternal and gestational weight gain, and (5) a range of approaches that promote appropriate weight during and after pregnancy. The final chapter describes cross-cutting themes that emerged from the workshop presentations and discussions.

REFERENCES

Flegal, K.M., Carroll, M.D., Ogden, C.L., and Johnson, C.L.
  2002   Prevalence and trends in obesity among U.S. adults, 1999–2000. *Journal of the American Medical Association* 288(14):1723–1727.
Hedley, A.A., Ogden, C.L., Johnson, C.L., Carroll, M.D., Curtin, L.R., and Flegal, K.M.
  2004   Prevalence of overweight and obesity among U.S. children, adolescents, and adults, 1999–2002. *Journal of the American Medical Association* 291(23):2847–2850.
Institute of Medicine
  1990   *Nutrition During Pregnancy.* Washington, DC: National Academy Press.
  1991   *Nutrition During Lactation.* Washington, DC: National Academy Press.
  1992   *Nutrition During Pregnancy and Lactation: An Implementation Guide.* Washington, DC: National Academy Press.
March of Dimes
  2004   *Maternal Obesity and Pregnancy: Weight Matters.* Available: http://www.marchofdimes.com/files/MP_MaternalObesity040605.pdf. [accessed August 14, 2006].
National Center for Health Statistics
  2004   *National Health and Nutrition Examination Survey, 1999–2002.* Available: http://www.cdc.gov/nchs/pressroom/04facts/obesity.htm. [accessed August 3, 2006].
National Heart, Lung, and Blood Institute
  1998   *Clinical Guidelines on the Identification, Evaluation, and Treatment of Overweight and Obesity in Adults.* (National Institutes of Health Publication 98-4083). Washington, DC: National Institutes of Health.
National Research Council
  1970   *Maternal Nutrition and the Course of Pregnancy.* Washington, DC: National Academy Press.
Ogden, C.L., Carroll, M.D., Curtin, L.R., McDowell, M.A., Tabak, C.J., and Flegal, K.M.
  2006   Prevalence of overweight and obesity in the United States, 1999–2004. *Journal of the American Medical Association* 295(13):1549–1555.

2

Trends in Maternal
and Gestational Weight

Mary Cogswell and Patricia Dietz described several important trends that have occurred in the weight distribution of different populations of women in their childbearing years. Figure 2-1 and Figure 2-2 summarize obesity and overweight prevalence trends among women of childbearing age (ages 20–39) and adolescents (ages 12–19) from 1960 to 2004, respectively. While several major sources provide data that help describe these trends, a national surveillance system for assessing maternal weight (prior to, during, and after pregnancy) does not exist. Available data sets have well-known shortcomings, but together they provide a general picture of the current situation with respect to maternal and gestational weight.

Among U.S. women ages 20 to 39 years who are not pregnant, the prevalence of obesity has increased from about 9 percent in 1970 to about 28 percent in 2000 (Flegal et al., 2002; Ogden et al., 2006). The obesity rate varies, however, among different ethnic populations: 24 percent for non-Hispanic white women, 36 percent for Mexican American women, and 50 percent for non-Hispanic black women (Ogden et al., 2006). Figure 2-3 summarizes these obesity prevalence rates in women of childbearing ages (ages 20–39). Adolescent girls (ages 12–19) have a prevalence of overweight (defined as greater than or equal to the 95th percentile of body mass index, BMI, based on gender and age) that statistically increased from 5 percent in 1970 to 15 percent in 2000. This rate increased slightly to 16 percent in 2004 (Flegal et al., 2002; Ogden et al., 2002, 2006). This prevalence was 15 percent for non-Hispanic white girls, 14 percent for Mexican

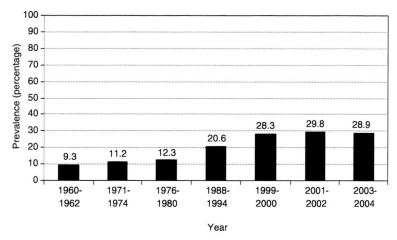

FIGURE 2-1 Prevalence (%) of obesity among nonpregnant U.S. women, ages 20–39. Obesity is defined as a body mass index of greater than 30.0.
SOURCE: Flegal et al. (2002) and Ogden et al. (2006).

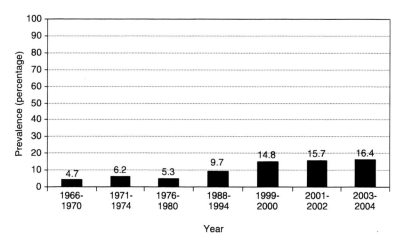

FIGURE 2-2 Prevalence (%) of overweight among nonpregnant U.S. adolescents, ages 12–19. Overweight is defined as greater than or equal to the 95th percentile of body mass index based on gender and age.
SOURCE: Ogden et al. (2002, 2006).

American girls, and 25 percent for non-Hispanic black girls (Ogden et al., 2006). Figure 2-4 summarizes these prevalence rates for overweight in adolescent women (ages 12–19). No nationally representative data exist for other minority populations, such as non-Mexican Hispanic, American Indian, Alaskan Native, and Asian women.

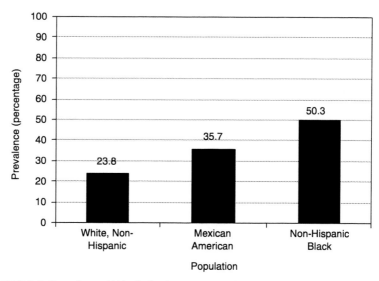

FIGURE 2-3 Prevalence (%) of obesity among U.S. nonpregnant women, ages 20–39, by race/ethnicity, 2003–2004. Obesity is defined as a body mass index of greater than 30.0.
SOURCE: Ogden et al. (2006).

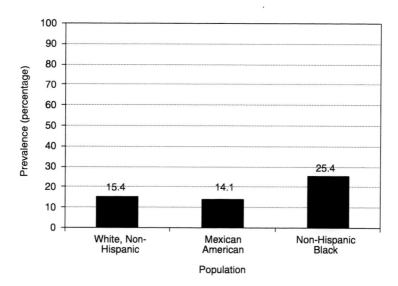

FIGURE 2-4 Prevalence (%) of overweight among U.S. nonpregnant women, ages 12–19, by race/ethnicity, 2003–2004. Overweight is defined as greater than or equal to the 95th percentile of body mass index based on gender and age.
SOURCE: Ogden et al. (2006).

PREPREGNANCY WEIGHT

Cogswell and Dietz observed that two sets of criteria exist for categorizing pregnancy weight status: the criteria of the 1990 Institute of Medicine (IOM) report and the 1998 criteria of the National Heart, Lung, and Blood Institute (NHLBI) (see Table 2-1). Studies that examined the association between prepregnancy BMI and maternal morbidity and mortality frequently classify prepregnant weight status by the IOM or NHLBI criteria.

These variations in the classification criteria have several ramifications, which can be seen in studies that draw on data from the Pregnancy and Nutrition Surveillance System (PNSS), a national database based on information about low-income women from 25 states and 6 tribal agencies. Estimates of the prevalence of underweight according to the IOM criteria using these data are more than twice the prevalence rates based on the NHLBI criteria. The prevalence of overweight is 40 percent lower and the prevalence of obesity is just slightly higher using IOM criteria. The prevalence of prepregnancy underweight using IOM criteria has declined from 22 percent in 1983 to about 12 percent in 2004, whereas the prevalence of overweight has increased from 24 percent in 1983 to 43 percent in 2004 (Centers for Disease Control and Prevention, 2006; see Figure 2-5).

GESTATIONAL WEIGHT GAIN

The recommendations of the 1990 IOM report specify weight gain ranges during pregnancy for singleton term births based on prepregnancy BMI (Table 2-2). National birth certificate data include maternal weight. However, data allow for a comparison between very low gestational weight gain groups (less than 15 lbs.) and very high gestational weight gain groups

TABLE 2-1 Criteria for Classifications of Prepregnancy Weight Status

	IOM (1990) Body Mass Index	NHLBI (1998) Body Mass Index
Underweight	<19.8	<18.5
Normal	19.8–26.0	18.5–24.9
Overweight	>26.0–29.0	25.0–29.9
Obese	>29.0	30.0+

SOURCE: Institute of Medicine (1990); National Heart, Lung, and Blood Institute (1998).

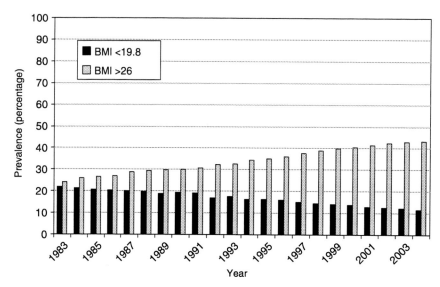

FIGURE 2-5 Prevalence of prepregnancy underweight (BMI <19.8) and overweight (BMI >26), Pregnancy and Nutrition Surveillance System. BMI refers to body mass index.
SOURCE: Centers for Disease Control and Prevention (2006).

TABLE 2-2 Summary of IOM Recommended Total Weight Gain Ranges for Pregnant Women,[a] by Prepregnancy Body Mass Index (BMI)[b]

Weight-for-Height Category	Recommended Total Gain	
	kg	lb
Low (BMI <19.8)	12.5–18	28–40
Normal (BMI of 19.8 to 26. 0)	11.5–16	25–35
High[c] (BMI >26.0 to 29.0)	7–11.5	15–25

[a]Young adolescents and black women should strive for gains at the upper end of the recommended range. Short women (<157 cm, or 62 in) should strive for gains at the lower end of the range.
[b]BMI is calculated using metric units.
[c]The recommended target weight gain for obese women (BMI >29.0) is at least 6.8 kg (15 lbs).

SOURCE: Institute of Medicine (1990).

(greater than 40 lbs.). Data are not available to support analyses of national birth certificate data in relation to the 1990 IOM recommendations based on prepregnancy BMI; such analyses can examine only total gestational weight gain at this time.

On the basis of these data, between 1990 and 2003, the percentage of women who gained less than 15 lbs. during pregnancy increased slightly from about 4 to 6 percent, and the percentage of women who gained more than 40 lbs. also increased, from 20 to about 25 percent (see Figure 2-6).

Weight Gain Across BMI Categories

Cogswell and Dietz described several data sets that make it possible to examine gestational weight gain across BMI categories (albeit not in nationally representative populations), including the National Vital Statistics System: Birth Data (NVSS), the Pregnancy Risk Assessment Monitoring System (PRAMS), the Pregnancy Nutrition Surveillance System (PNSS), and the California Maternal and Infant Health Assessment (CA-MIHA) (Table 2-3). These data sets support analyses of the distribution of gestational weight among different age groups as well as selected racial and ethnic populations (see Table 2-4).

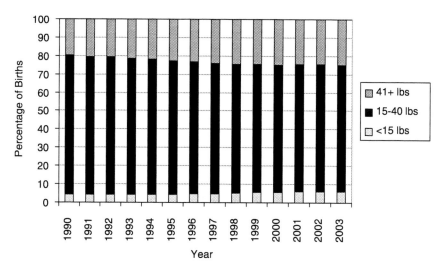

FIGURE 2-6 U.S. trends in weight gain during pregnancy, singleton, term, primiparous births, 1990–2003.
SOURCE: 1990–2000: Rhodes et al. (2003), reproduced with permission from *Pediatrics*, 111:1181–1185; 2001–2003: National Vital Statistics System, birth data, unpublished analysis.

TABLE 2-3 U.S. Data Sources for Gestational Weight Distribution

Sources	Description
National Vital Statistics System: Birth Data	Contains data on all births in the United States as reported on state birth certificates
Pregnancy Risk Assessment Monitoring System	State-specific population-based surveys of mother's attitudes and experiences before, during, and after pregnancy • Linked to birth certificates • Currently collecting data in 39 states (although data for the past 10 years are available only in 9 states) • Height and prepregnancy weight are self-reported • Weight gain during pregnancy is from the birth certificate
Pregnancy Nutrition Surveillance Systems	Program-based public health surveillance system among low-income pregnant women who participated in federally funded public health programs • Currently collects data from programs in 25 states and 6 trial agencies • Height and weight at first prenatal visit measured by clinician • Prepregnancy weight and weight gain during pregnancy are self-reported
California Maternal and Infant Health Assessment	Ongoing population-based survey of mothers delivering live infants in California from February through May of each year • All indicators are self-reported

SOURCE: Cogswell, Dietz, and Branum (2006).

Cogswell and Dietz presented preliminary analyses of these data sets. Their analyses indicate that similar gestational weight gain patterns can be found across the different data sets, with several exceptions. The PNSS data set (which includes more minority populations) shows higher estimates (of about 5 percent) for women who gained less than 15 lbs. during their pregnancies. PNSS also shows a higher percentage of women who have gained more than 40 lbs. during their pregnancies than other data sources.

These data sets also contain data for BMI. In the PRAMS data from 1993 to 2003, the gestational weight gains of a little over one-third of women were consistent with the 1990 IOM recommendations, with no real change evident over time. In the CA-MIHA data from 1999 to 2004, about 40 percent of women met the IOM recommendations for weight gain during pregnancy, with little change over time. And in the PNSS data from 1992 to 2004, the weight gains during pregnancy of about one-third of women were within the IOM guidelines. In addition, the PNSS data suggest

TABLE 2-4 Distributions of Age and Race/Ethnicity by Data Source, Current Year

	NVSS (%)	PRAMS (%)	PNSS (%)	CA-MIHA (%)
Age (years)				
<20	10	10	18	8
20–34	73	75	75	75
35+	17	15	7	17
Race/Ethnicity				
Non-Hispanic white	62	64	50	35
Non-Hispanic black	15	15	24	5
Hispanic	18	15	22	45
Other	5	6	4	14

NOTES: NVSS = National Vital Statistics System: Birth Data; PRAMS = Pregnancy Risk Assessment Monitoring System; PNSS = Pregnancy and Nutrition Surveillance System; CA-MIHA = California Maternal and Infant Health Assessment.
SOURCE: Cogswell, Dietz, and Branum (2006).

a general increase in the percentage of women gaining weight during pregnancy above the IOM recommendations, from about 37 percent in 1993 to about 46 percent in 2004, and a decrease in the percentage of women gaining weight during pregnancy below the IOM guidelines, from about 30 to 23 percent also in 1993–2004.

Age, Race/Ethnicity, and Stature

The 1990 IOM report provided specific gestational weight gain recommendations for particular subgroups, including adolescents, members of racial and ethnic groups, women of short stature, and women carrying twins. Data collected since 1990 allow for an examination of the degree to which these recommendations are consistent with gestational weight patterns among different age groups and racial and ethnic populations. Analyses of the PNSS data reveal gestational weight gain distributions for younger adolescents that are similar to the distribution of women of other ages. Similar analyses of the PRAMS data show that similar proportions of black and white women gain at the upper half of the IOM recommendations, about 20 percent, a finding consistent with the PNSS data, although at a lower percentage (about 12 to 13 percent).

The 1990 IOM report recommended that women of short stature (less than 62 inches tall) should strive for gestational weight gains in the lower end of the recommended gestational weight gain for their BMI. Analyses of the PNSS data, however, indicate that such women were no more likely to be in the lower half of the IOM recommendations than taller women, a finding consistent with analyses of the PRAMS data.

In summary, analyses of the national data sets suggest that approximately one-third of pregnant women gain within the IOM gestational weight gain guidelines and that weight gain pregnancy patterns have been fairly stable over time, except in the PNSS, which contains more low-income women. There is no evidence that the IOM recommendations for specific populations of women have been followed.

POSTPARTUM WEIGHT RETENTION

As the speakers' overview of the distribution of maternal weight indicated, national data on postpartum BMI or weight retention after pregnancy are limited. Analyses of data from the 1988 National Child and Infant Health Survey suggest that, on average at 12 months postpartum, about 40 percent of women in the sample retained 14 lbs. above their prepregnancy weight status. Obese women (BMI >29) were excluded from these analyses since the IOM gestational weight gain recommendations do not set an upper weight gain limit, and gestational weight gain was categorized using the IOM classification criteria. In this study, black women retained more weight postpartum than white women in all BMI categories. In addition, black women who had higher rates of weight gain during pregnancy were also likely to retain more weight postpartum. This pattern was similar to white women who gained in excess of the IOM recommendations (Figure 2-7). A discussion panelist, Anna Marie Siega-Riz, indicated that her unpublished study of a shorter period (3 months postpartum) found that the average amount of weight retained postpartum was about 9 lbs. with 45 percent of white women and 57 percent of black women retaining more than 10 lbs.

National data on postpartum weight retention collected since the 1990 IOM recommendations have not been analyzed. There are, however, some national and state data sources that may provide useful information about postpartum weight retention status since the IOM recommendations. For example, the 1988 National Maternal and Infant Health Survey data indicate that gestational weight gain is associated with excess postpartum weight retention (Keppel and Taffel, 1993), and preliminary analyses of the Early Childhood Longitudinal Study Birth Cohort suggest that little association exists between gestational weight gain and postpartum obesity except for women who weighed 130 to 149 lbs. before pregnancy. Other data sources include the Infant Feeding Practices Survey-2 (for which data are not yet available) and limited data from the PNSS (Table 2-5).

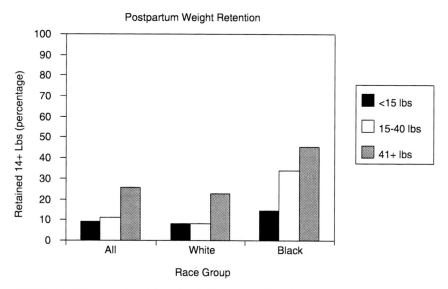

FIGURE 2-7 Retained weight after delivery (14+ lbs), by gestational weight gain in reference to IOM recommendations, United States, 1988 (excludes women with BMI >29).
SOURCE: Adapted with permission from Keppel and Taffel (1993).

TABLE 2-5 U.S. Data Sources to Determine Postpartum Weight Distribution

Sources	Description
Early Childhood Longitudinal Study Birth Cohort	A nationally representative longitudinal study of U.S. children born in 2001 that looks at children's health, development, care, and education from birth through first grade
Infant Feeding Practices Survey-2	A national mail panel survey on infant feeding practices that enrolled pregnant women in 2005
Pregnancy Nutrition Surveillance System	Program-based public health surveillance system that monitors risk factors associated with infant mortality and poor birth outcomes among low-income pregnant women who participate in federally funded public health programs, 1983+ (1988+ for pregnancy weight gain)

SOURCE: Cogswell, Dietz, and Branum (2006).

SUMMARY

The workshop presentations indicated that almost 30 percent of women of childbearing age (20–39 years) are obese, and the prevalence of obesity is even higher among Mexican American and non-Hispanic black women. Over 15 percent of adolescent girls (ages 12–19) are overweight, with higher prevalence rates among non-Hispanic black adolescents. No national surveillance system exists to adequately monitor maternal weight prior to, during, and after pregnancy. The limited data that are available from 1983 through 2004, prepregnancy underweight declined, while the prevalence of prepregnancy overweight increased. The numbers of women gaining less than 15 and more than 40 lbs. during pregnancy (between 1990 and 2003) have slightly increased between 1990 and 2003. Postpartum weight retention data are limited, although data from 1998 indicate that black women retained more weight than white women in all BMI categories.

During the presentations and discussion sessions, several challenges were addressed for the prevention of obesity among adolescent girls and women of childbearing age and for the promotion of healthy weight gain during pregnancy. They include the striking absence of evidence of increased adherence to the IOM gestational weight gain recommendations during the course of a pregnancy among general or selected populations of women and the variations in prevalence estimates that persist from the use of different classification criteria (IOM or NHLBI). As noted by the participants, there continues to be uncertainty as to which criteria are best for categorizing prepregnant overweight and obesity. Finally, there is uncertainty concerning the application of the adult criteria (prepregnancy BMI and gestational weight gain recommendations), which are based on an assumption of relatively static adult weight (exclusive of pregnancy), to categorize adolescents in studies of weight-related pregnancy outcomes.

REFERENCES

Centers for Disease Control and Prevention
  2006   *Pediatric and Pregnancy Nutrition Surveillance System. Pregnancy Data Tables.* Available: http://www.cdc.gov/pednss/pnss_tables/tables_numeric.htm. [accessed August 3, 2006].
Cogswell, M.E., Dietz, P.M., and Branum, A.M.
  2006   Maternal Weight, Before, During, and After Pregnancy in the United States. Presentation at the Workshop on the Impact of Pregnancy Weight on Maternal and Child Health, May 30, Washington, DC.
Flegal, K.M., Carroll, M.D., Ogden, C.L., and Johnson, C.L.
  2002   Prevalence and trends in obesity among U.S. adults, 1999–2000. *Journal of the American Medical Association* 288(14):1723–1727.
Institute of Medicine
  1990   *Nutrition During Pregnancy.* Washington, DC: National Academy Press.

Keppel, K.G., and Taffel, S.M.
   1993   Pregnancy-related weight gain and retention: Implications of the 1990 Institute of Medicine guidelines. *American Journal of Public Health* 83(8):1100–1103.
Ogden, C.L., Carroll, M.D., Curtin, L.R., McDowell, M.A., Tabak, C.J., and Flegal, K.M.
   2006   Prevalence of overweight and obesity in the United States, 1999–2004. *Journal of the American Medical Association* 295(13):1549–1555.
Ogden, C.L., Flegal, K.M., Carroll, M.D., and Johnson, C.L.
   2002   Prevalence and trends in overweight among U.S. children and adolescents, 1999–2000. *Journal of the American Medical Association* 288(14):1728–1732.
National Heart, Lung, and Blood Institute
   1998   *Clinical Guidelines on the Identification, Evaluation, and Treatment of Overweight and Obesity in Adults.* (National Institutes of Health Publication 98-4083). Washington, DC: National Institutes of Health.
Rhodes, J.C., Schoendorf, K.C., and Parker, J.D.
   2003   Contributions of excess weight gain during pregnancy and macrosomia to the cesarean delivery rate, 1990–2000. *Pediatrics* 111(5 Part 2):1181–1185.

3

Determinants of
Gestational Weight Gain

Determinants of gestational weight gain include a range of biological, metabolic, and social factors. Several workshop speakers discussed the base of knowledge and current understanding of the complicated relationship between biological and social factors in determining gestational weight gain. In addition, they indicated how this research could provide insight on factors that may impede or foster compliance with the recommended guidelines for gestation weight gain. This chapter is framed by speakers at the workshop; distinguishing between biological factors and social factors poses a significant challenge as knowledge is gained about the nature of their interactions. Many processes involve both components.

GESTATIONAL WEIGHT GAIN

Janet King observed that gestational weight gain includes three components: (1) the products of conception (i.e., the fetus, placenta, and amniotic fluid), (2) maternal tissues (i.e., uterus, mammary, and blood), and (3) maternal fat reserves. The fat reserves comprise about 30 percent of the total gain on average. The components of gain can also be divided into water, about 65 percent of the total, fat, about 30 percent and the most variable, and protein, the remaining 5 percent (Butte et al., 2003; Hytten and Chamberlain, 1980; Kopp-Hoolihan et al., 1999).

Recommended Gestational Weight Gain

The 1990 Institute of Medicine (IOM) report *Nutrition During Pregnancy* recommended guidelines for gestational weight gain. To derive the recommendations, gestational weight gain was summarized for women in different prepregnancy body mass index (BMI) groups giving birth to infants weighing between 6.6 and 8.8 lbs., which was considered the normal range of infant birth weight with good outcomes. The range of reported gestational weight gain, which was extremely wide, was then narrowed by the committee to the resultant IOM recommendations (Table 2-2). Abrams and Parker (1990) reported the mean gestational weight gains of women with good outcomes (i.e., infants with birth weights within the normal range) in very similar BMI groups to those used by the IOM committee. The gestational weight gains of women in the underweight and normal-weight groups were generally consistent with the IOM recommendations, but the gains of overweight and obese women exceeded the recommendations. Wells et al. (2006) reported the odds ratio of gaining either above or below the IOM's recommended range was high in women with a pre-pregnancy BMI greater than 29 compared with women with prepregnancy BMI of 19.8 to 26—an odds ratio of 19 of gaining above and nearly 7 of gaining below.

Recommended Rate of Gestational Weight Gain

The 1990 IOM committee also recommended a rate of weight gain during pregnancy to facilitate the clinical monitoring of weight changes in pregnant women (Institute of Medicine, 1990). The recommendations were based on data from the 1980 National Natality Survey. For normal-weight women, a gain of about 0.9 lb/week in the second and third trimesters was suggested; overweight or obese women were advised to gain slightly less and underweight women slightly more. Studies of rates of gestational weight gain show that women deviate considerably from these recommendations. Data from over 113,000 women in the Pregnancy Risk Assessment Monitoring System (PRAMS) showed that very low rates of gain (<0.26 lb/week) were more prevalent for obese and very obese women, 8 and 19 percent, respectively, than in underweight and normal-weight women, 2 percent in both groups (Dietz et al., 2006). About 10 percent of the women gained weight at twice the recommended weight (more than >1.7 lbs/week).

Pattern of Gestational Weight Gain

Studies of the pattern of gestational weight gain help to determine when the greatest rate of gain occurs and how it varies with maternal prepregnancy BMI. Both Butte et al. (2003) and Carmichael et al. (1997) reported greater rates of weight gain in the second trimester compared with the third, with lower average rates in overweight or obese women. However, the pattern of gain differed in a study of 1,367 Filipino women who started pregnancy weighing less than the typical American woman (Siega-Riz and Adair, 1993). Underweight women (BMI <18.5) gained more weight during pregnancy than normal-weight or overweight women due to higher gains in the first trimester. Overweight women (BMI >25) lost a small amount of weight in the first trimester, but they gained at a more rapid rate in the third trimester, when fetal growth rates are the highest. In sum, King observed, studies suggest that the rate of maternal weight gain during the first half of pregnancy, when fat stores are accumulating, tends to be lower in women with higher amounts of fat stores at conception. Also, the average rate of weight gain during pregnancy among U.S. women is greater than the 0.9 lb./week recommended by the 1990 IOM report.

BIOLOGICAL AND METABOLIC FACTORS OF GESTATIONAL WEIGHT GAIN

King provided an overview of the role of biological and metabolic factors in gestational weight gain. Studies of the influence of biological and metabolic factors tend to be cross-sectional and observational, with relatively small sample sizes. Although it is difficult to draw any conclusions about the link between these factors and gestational weight gain, two themes emerge from the research conducted to date: (1) interactions among several biological factors (i.e., prepregnancy weight, age, parity, and stature) influence gestational weight gain and (2) the biological influences on gestational weight gain vary widely among women. Other potential metabolic factors that may affect gestational weight gain (i.e., placental secretions or metabolic changes in obese women) remain poorly understood.

Prepregnancy Body Mass Index

In 1990, the IOM committee concluded that maternal prepregnancy BMI is a primary determinant of gestational weight gain and referenced all of its recommendations to prepregnancy BMI (Institute of Medicine, 1990). Research studies presented at the workshop continue to support this conclusion.

Maternal Age

The effect of maternal age on gestational weight gain has been studied almost exclusively in young (adolescent) mothers; no data from older mothers were located. Three new studies of gestational weight gain in adolescents have been published since the IOM report was released in 1990 (Hediger et al., 1990; Johnston et al., 1991; Stevens-Simon et al., 1993). As reported in the 1990 IOM report, these studies suggest that the ratio of infant birth weight to maternal gestational weight gain tends to be lower among adolescents than adults, and higher gestational weight gains do not improve birth weight in infants born to adolescent mothers. One study has reported higher rates of total gestational weight gain among adolescent mothers than among adults (Hediger et al., 1990).

Parity

The 1990 IOM report reported that multiparous women tend to gain less weight than primiparous women (i.e., first-time mothers). A comprehensive study of 523 women in the United Kingdom confirmed this finding (Harris et al., 1997). In addition, two studies found that high parity is associated with a higher BMI later in life due to weight retention following each pregnancy (Harris et al., 1997; Wolfe et al., 1997). As mentioned in the previous section, higher prepregnancy BMI is the primary determinant of gestational weight gain. King described one study of U.S. women that found ethnic variations in the relationship between parity and body weight (Wolfe et al., 1997). In this study, black women who were underweight at conception tend to retain about twice as much weight following a pregnancy than do underweight white women. Elizabeth McAnarney noted that young primiparous adolescents are at particular risk for greater weight gain (Howie et al., 2003).

Stature

Data on the effect of maternal height on gestational weight gain are very limited. In 1990, the IOM committee reported that short women (<62 in) tend to gain less than taller (>67 in) women (Institute of Medicine, 1990). In a study of 4,791 Hispanic women living in Los Angeles, short stature (<62 in) increased the risk of poor total weight gain by 50 percent among underweight and normal-weight women, but not among overweight or obese women (Siega-Riz and Hobel, 1997). The interactions among maternal prepregnancy BMI status and stature in affecting gestational weight gain need further evaluation.

Determinants of Maternal Fat Gain

Fat gain is the most variable of the three components (water, fat, and protein) of maternal weight gain. The amount of fat gained is more strongly associated with total weight gain than any other component (Butte et al., 2003; Kopp-Hoolihan et al., 1999). It also is the component of gestational weight gain that contributes to higher BMI later in life. For example, in a small study of 10 women who were similar in terms of race/ethnicity, weight status at conception, and parity, maternal body fat changes varied from a small loss to a gain of over 22 lbs. (Kopp-Hoolihan et al., 1999).

Although maternal total energy intake undoubtedly influences maternal fat gain, other biological regulators, such as genetics, insulin, and leptin, probably also play a role. Studies show that maternal genotype influences total weight and, presumably, fat gain. For example, one study found that women who are homozygous for the T allele of the G-protein β_3 subunit gain statistically more weight during pregnancy than women with other alleles (Dishy et al., 2003). In another study, polymorphisms of the PPAR-$\gamma 2$ gene increased weight gain during pregnancy in women with gestational diabetes (Tok et al., 2006). Circulating levels of the hormones insulin and leptin are also associated with excessive amounts of weight gain. In one study, women in the highest quartile for fasting insulin concentrations when they registered for prenatal care had a twofold increased risk for excessive gestational weight gain and a 3.6-fold increased risk of excess weight retained postpartum, suggesting that the excess weight gained was fat (Scholl and Chen, 2002). Higher leptin concentrations at entry for prenatal care have also been found to be associated with excess weight retained postpartum; for each increase in the log of the initial leptin concentration, weight retention increased by 16 lbs. (Stein et al., 1998).

Summary of Biological Predictors

In 1990 the IOM concluded that prepregnancy BMI was a direct determinant of gestational weight gain (Institute of Medicine, 1990). Studies conducted during the intervening 15 years support that conclusion, and also advance understanding of other biological and metabolic factors that may moderate that relationship. Maternal biological factors, such as age, parity, and stature, along with maternal genetic and metabolic state, appear to influence the amount and composition of weight gain.[1] The role of other potential metabolic factors that may affect gestational weight gain—such as genetics and hormonal regulators that affect metabolism—remain poorly understood. Future research is needed to identify these factors and to untangle the complex relationships between biological factors and gestational weight gain.

SOCIAL PREDICTORS OF GESTATIONAL WEIGHT GAIN

Naomi Stotland provided an overview of a large body of literature on social predictors of gestational weight gain, including studies from the 1990

---

[1]It is important to note that other determinants not presented in the workshop may also exist.

IOM report as well as subsequent analyses. This research describes predictors of both inadequate and excessive weight gain. The 1990 report focused on predictors of inadequate gestational weight gain, but more recent attention has focused on predictors of excessive gestational weight gain as a result of concern over obesity.

Multiple Predictors

Recent studies have attempted to isolate social predictors of gestational weight gain by using large samples and collecting measures of multiple potential predictors. Siega-Riz and Hobel (1997) looked specifically at predictors of gestational weight gain below the IOM guidelines in a Hispanic population. For women with low or normal prepregnancy weight, none of the social factors they considered was associated with increased risk of, or actual, insufficient gestational weight gain, but several factors were associated with decreased risk. Among women with low or normal weight, being U.S.-born, being primiparous, being under age 29, having a planned pregnancy, and having a close relative die during the pregnancy decreased the risk of insufficient gestational weight gain. Among the subgroup of women who were overweight or obese at the start of their pregnancies, however, a history of physical abuse increased the risk of low gestational weight gain. Financial support from the fathers of the babies also decreased the risk of low gestational weight gain in this sample.

In a study of mostly black and white participants in the Special Supplemental Nutrition Program for Women, Infants, and Children (WIC), Hickey et al. (1999) found that a short interpregnancy interval, smoking, and late entry into prenatal care were all associated with insufficient gestational weight gain. These associations, however, varied by race/ethnicity and by prepregnancy BMI.

Olson and Strawderman (2003) found that change in the amount of food intake from prepregnancy to pregnancy, change in physical activity from prepregnancy to pregnancy, and smoking behaviors were independently associated with gestational weight gain. Finally, Wells et al. (2006) used PRAMS data from Colorado to show that insufficient gestational weight gain was associated with underweight and obesity, rural residence, low education, and smoking. Excessive gestational weight gain was associated with overweight and obesity and 12 or fewer years of education.

Individual Predictors

Stotland indicated that numerous studies have examined a wide range of individual characteristics to find possible predictors of gestational weight gain. These include education and socioeconomic status; work and physical activity; caloric intake; overall health status; smoking, alcohol intake, and substance use; eating disorders; unintended pregnancy; domestic violence; and provider advice. The research on each of these factors is reviewed below.

Education and Socioeconomic Status

Two studies of educational status suggest that lower education is associated with increased risk of insufficient gestational weight gain (Hickey et al., 1999; Wells et al., 2006). Examining socioeconomic status (SES) is more complicated because studies looking at social predictors tend to use cohorts of low-income women only, allowing for little variation in SES. In their study, Olson and Strawderman (2003) reported that women with a family income less than 185 percent of the poverty line were about 2.6 times more likely to have excessive weight gains during pregnancy than women with higher incomes. For the overweight and obese subgroup in the Hispanic cohort studied by Siega-Riz and Hobel (1997), receiving financial support from the baby's father decreased the risk of insufficient gain during pregnancy. The Colorado PRAMS study (Wells et al., 2006) found no association between SES and the risk of either insufficient or excessive gain during pregnancy. However, the women most at risk, those with no prenatal care, may not be represented in these surveys.

Work and Physical Activity

Work and physical activity were linked to pregnancy outcomes (e.g., low birth weight, prematurity) but not maternal weight in the 1990 IOM report. Data since 1990 are conflicting, generally showing either no difference in gestational weight gain among women with varying amounts of physical activity or showing decreased gain in women with higher physical activity. Two meta-analyses examining a set of heterogeneous studies reported no overall difference in gestational weight gain by physical activity. However, a set of smaller studies has reported reduced gestational weight gain in women who exercised when compared with nonrandomized controls. And Olson and Strawderman (2003) found that decreased self-reported physical activity was associated with excessive gestational weight gain.

Caloric Intake

Before the 1990 IOM report, most studies of caloric intake during pregnancy were supplementation trials conducted in developing countries. These studies generally showed that supplementation resulted in increased gestational weight gain. A number of observational studies of caloric intake have generally supported this relationship. Olson and Strawderman (2003) used a proxy measure for energy intake by questioning women about changes in the amount of food eaten prior to and during pregnancy. They found that women who ate "much more" during than before their pregnancy had an adjusted odds ratio of 2.35 for excessive weight gain during pregnancy. In a recent prospective observational study conducted in Iceland, Olafsdottir et al. (2006) surveyed a cohort of 406 women with a semiquantitative questionnaire about food frequency that was completed during the women's second and third trimesters. A higher energy intake in late pregnancy was associated with a lower risk of insufficient gestational weight gain and a higher risk of excessive gestational gain. The researchers also considered both overall energy intake and change in energy intake between the first and second survey points. They found that excessive gain was associated with increased energy intake during that time period, but absolute energy intake in early pregnancy was not associated with gestational weight gain.[2]

Beyond general food intake, recent studies have also examined consumption of different types of food as well as macronutrient intake. In the Iceland study, the investigators also found that consumption of dairy products and sweets in late pregnancy was associated with a decreased risk of inadequate gain and an increased risk of excessive gain during pregnancy (Olafsdottir et al., 2006). The study by Olson and Strawderman (2003) found that women who consumed three or more servings of fruits and vegetables a day gained 1.81 lbs. less than women who consumed fewer than three servings. A study of adolescents by Stevens-Simon and McAnarney (1992) showed that those who consumed fewer than three snacks a day had slower weight gain during pregnancy.

In a small randomized clinical trial of a low-glycemic versus a high-glycemic diet, Clapp (2002) found that the women on the low-glycemic diet gained less weight during pregnancy (22.9 compared with 40.9 lbs.).[3] However, Siega-Riz and Hobel (1997), examining the associations between the glycemic load, race/ethnicity, and gestational weight gain in their cohort of 2,000 pregnant women in North Carolina, reported no statistical effect of

---

[2]Overall energy intake is an absolute measure of calories consumed, regardless of whether this amount is consistent over time or inconsistent; an increase in energy intake indicates a change in energy intake between two points in time, without regard to the absolute level of intake at either time.

[3]Glycemic index is a numerical system of measuring how much of a rise in circulating blood glucose a carbohydrate triggers, for example, consumption of high-glycemic index foods results in higher and more rapid increases in blood glucose levels than the consumption of low-glycemic index foods.

glycemic load[4] alone on gestational weight gain. Moreover, they also found that race/ethnicity was associated with prepregnancy weight. During the workshop discussion, Siega-Riz suggested that race/ethnicity may interact with glycemic processes, since in her study white women with higher glycemic load increases are more sensitive to increased weight gain during pregnancy, although this was not true for black women. The Icelandic study found that the percentage of energy intake from various macronutrients is an important predictor of weight gain only among overweight women and late in pregnancy (Olafsdottir et al., 2006). Women who had insufficient gestational weight gain had a lower percentage intake from fat and a higher percentage intake from carbohydrates than women who had optimal or excessive gains.

Overall Health Status

Few studies consider overall health status and gestational weight gain. One study found that chronic or gestational diabetes was associated with increased risk of insufficient gestational weight gain (Brawarsky et al., 2005).

Smoking, Alcohol, and Substance Use

Most studies of smoking published since the 1990 IOM report show an increased risk of inadequate gestational weight gain associated with tobacco use (Furuno et al., 2004; Olson and Strawderman, 2003; Wells et al., 2006). An additional study noted by Calvin Hobel found that smoking status may contribute to the association of parity and the risk of becoming overweight, in that, among smokers, increased risk of high BMI later in life is not associated with parity (Gunderson et al., 2005). Most studies since 1990 of alcohol and illegal substance use show either no association between alcohol use and gestational weight gain or slightly higher gains among drinkers, including adolescents (Stevens-Simon and McAnarney, 1992).

Eating Disorders

Few studies consider eating disorders and gestational weight gain. One study found no overall difference in gestational weight gain of women with eating disorders compared with a control group, although the anorexic subgroup had a statistically lower mean gain than the controls (Kouba et al., 2005).

---

[4]Glycemic load describes the quality (glycemic index) and quantity of carbohydrate in a meal or diet.

Unintended Pregnancy

Data concerning the effect of unintended pregnancy on gestational weight gain are somewhat conflicting. Hickey et al. (1997) found that mistimed or unplanned pregnancy was associated with an increased risk (adjusted odds ratio) for insufficient gestational weight gain among black women. In the study by Siega-Riz and Hobel (1997), planned pregnancy was associated with a marginally statistically significant decreased risk for insufficient gestational weight gain, but only among the low and normal-weight subjects in this Hispanic cohort. The PRAMS study has not found an association between gestational weight gain and planned pregnancy (Wells et al., 2006).

Domestic Violence

Two studies of domestic violence suggest an association between intimate partner violence, or domestic violence, and insufficient gestational weight gain (McFarlane et al., 1996; Siega-Riz and Hobel, 1997).

Provider Advice

Cogswell et al. (1999) examined the role of professional health care provider advice in influencing gestational weight gain through a mail survey of a predominantly white, middle-class cohort of women. The survey asked how much weight the women were told to gain by their health care provider during pregnancy, their target weight gains, and their actual gain. The study found that the advised and target gains were strongly correlated with actual weight gain. Receiving no advice on gestational weight gain, a fairly prevalent situation, was associated with weight gain outside the guidelines. Provider advice to gain below the IOM recommendations was associated with actual weight gain below the recommendations (an adjusted odds ratio of 3.6), and advice above the guidelines had the same odds ratio for higher rates of gain. The absence of professional health care advice concerning weight gain put women at risk for both too high and too low gains. In this study, black women were more likely to report receiving advice to gain less than the 1990 IOM recommendations.

Research Needs

The increasing prevalence of obesity emphasizes the need to shift focus to predictors of excessive gestational weight gain. The nature and source of provider advice intervention is a research area that could indicate how the role of provider and type of advice influence gestational weight gain.

Stotland highlighted a phenomenon called centering pregnancy or group prenatal care, which gives patients extended time with the provider in a group setting. Although group prenatal care can improve birth weight in women at risk for having low birth weight infants, virtually no research has examined how the type of prenatal care affects gestational weight gain.

Another promising area of future research, concerning the type of provider (midwife versus physician) of care, has not been examined. For example, studies have not yet examined differences between midwives and physicians in providing guidance on prenatal weight gain.

More research is also needed about maternal dietary factors, such as low-glycemic load diets and their association with gestational weight gain. A third area for future research is suggested by the consistent indication of interactions among social factors, race/ethnicity, and rates of gestational weight gain. The presence of such interactions suggests the need to study them further to elucidate the effects of specific social factors on a race/ethnicity or cultural group. The data are unclear and conflicting concerning the role of physical activity and exercise; more studies are needed of interventions, both during and prior to pregnancy, to improve physical activity. Other potential social factors that may affect gestational weight gain (e.g., hormonal contraception) also remain poorly understood.

Summary of Social Predictors

The initial predictors of gestational weight gain (insufficient or excessive) identified in the 1990 IOM report remain important, but more recent literature has identified several additional predictors, such as unintended pregnancy, eating disorders, physical activity provider advice, and diet. Some potential predictors have not yet been extensively explored (Table 3-1).

SUMMARY

The King and Stotland reviews of the contributions of biological/metabolic and social factors to both insufficient and excessive gestational weight gain suggest an intricate web of process and interaction. New data on the predictors of gestational weight gain remain limited in scope. Prepregnancy BMI remains the primary determinant of gestational weight gain, but other biological and metabolic factors probably moderate that relationship. Maternal biological factors, such as age, parity, and stature, along with maternal genetic and metabolic state, appear to influence both the amount and composition of gestational weight gain. Complex interactions among the biological factors influencing gestational weight gain vary widely among different populations of women. Future research could reveal the nature of

TABLE 3-1 Social Predictors of Inadequate and Excessive Gestational Weight Gain

Inadequate Gestational Weight Gain	Excessive Gestational Weight Gain
Identified in the IOM (1990) report: • Lower socioeconomic status/education • Cigarette smoking • Low energy intake • Use of illegal substances Identified since the 1990 report: • Low dairy intake • Unintended pregnancy • Domestic violence • Anorexia nervosa • Short interpregnancy interval • Lack of provider advice/advice less than the guidelines	Identified in the IOM (1990) report: • High energy intake • Increase in energy intake Identified since the 1990 report: • Decrease in physical activity • High-glycemic diet • High-fat diet • Consumption of sweets • Lack of provider advice/advice greater than the guidelines Possible predictors: • Type of provider[a] • Type of prenatal care[a]

NOTE: IOM = Institute of Medicine.

[a]Possible social predictors of gestational weight gain that have not been extensively explored.

SOURCE: Stotland (2006).

these complex interactions and their influence on the rate and pattern of weight gain during pregnancy.

Numerous social factors are predictors of either inadequate or excessive gestational weight gain. Key social predictors of gestational weight gain include smoking, SES, education, use of illegal substances, diet (which results in biological factors such as energy intake), physical activity, unintended pregnancy, domestic violence, eating disorders, and provider advice. In addition, the literature suggests other potential social predictors—type of provider and type of prenatal care—that deserve consideration. The literature on racial/ethnic differences in these biological and social predictors is limited.

This review of both biological and social factors of gestational weight gain illustrates factors that may impede or foster compliance with recommended gestational weight guidelines and may guide Title V maternal and child health programs in helping women of childbearing age to achieve and maintain recommended weight before, during, and after pregnancy. Recent research suggests that narrowing the range of recommended gestational weight gain values may be especially important for overweight or obese women. However, it is unclear whether women would respond to such a change, since a high proportion of women gain in excess of current recommended guidelines.

REFERENCES

Abrams, B., and Parker, J.D.
    1990   Maternal weight gain in women with good pregnancy outcome. *Obstetrics and Gynecology* 76:1–7.
Brawarsky, P., Stotland, N.E., Jackson, R.A., Fuentes-Afflick, E., Escobar, G.J., Rubashkin, N., and Haas, J.S.
    2005   Pre-pregnancy and pregnancy-related factors and the risk of excessive or inadequate gestational weight gain. *International Journal of Gynaecology and Obstetrics* 91(2):125–131.
Butte, N.F., Ellis, K.J., Wong, W.W., Hopkinson, J.M., and O'Brian Smith, E.
    2003   Composition of gestational weight gain impacts maternal fat retention and infant birth weight. *American Journal of Obstetrics and Gynecology* 189:1423–1432.
Carmichael, S., Abrams, B., and Selvin, S.
    1997   The pattern of maternal weight gain in women with good pregnancy outcomes. *American Journal of Public Health* 87:1984–1988.
Clapp, J.F. III.
    2002   Maternal carbohydrate intake and pregnancy outcome. *Proceedings of the Nutrition Society* 61(1):45–50.
Cogswell, M.E., Scanlon, K.S., Fein, S.B., and Schieve, L.A.
    1999   Medically advised, mother's personal target, and actual weight gain during pregnancy. *Obstetrics and Gynecology* 94(4):616–622.
Dietz, P.M., Callaghan, W.M., Cogswell, M.E., Morrow, B., Ferre, C., and Schieve, L.A.
    2006   Combined effects of prepregnancy body mass index and weight gain during pregnancy on the risk of preterm delivery. *Epidemiology* 17:170–177.
Dishy, V., Gupta, S., Landau, R., Xie, H.G., Kim, R.B., Smiley, R.M., Byrne, D.W., Wood, A.J., and Stein, C.M.
    2003   G-protein b3 subunits 825 C/T polymorphism is associated with weight gain during pregnancy. *Pharmacogenetics* 13:241–242.
Furuno, J.P., Gallicchio, L., and Sexton, M.
    2004   Cigarette smoking and low maternal weight gain in Medicaid-eligible pregnant women. *Journal of Women's Health* 13(7):770–777.
Gunderson, E.P., Quesenberry, C.P., Lewis, C.E., Tsai, A.L., Sternfeld, B., West, D.S., and Signey, S.
    2004   Development of overweight associated with childbearing depends on smoking habit: The Coronary Artery Risk Development in Young Adults (CARDIA) study. *Obesity Research* 12(12):2041–2053.
Harris, H.E., Ellison, G.T.H., and Holliday, M.
    1997   Is there an independent association between parity and maternal weight gain? *Annals of Human Biology* 24:507–591.
Hediger, M.L., School, T.O., Ances, I.G., Belsky, D.H., and Salmon, R.W.
    1990   Rate and amount of weight gain during adolescent pregnancy: Associations with maternal weight-for-height and birth weight. *American Journal of Clinical Nutrition* 52:793–799.
Hickey, C.A., Cliver, S.P., Goldenberg, R.L., McNeal, S.F., and Hoffman, H.J.
    1997   Low prenatal weight gain among low-income women: What are the risk factors? *Birth* 24(2):102–108.

Hickey, C.A., Kreauter, M., Bronstein, J., Johnson, V., McNeal, S.F., Harshbarger, D.S., and Woolbright, L.A.
1999   Low prenatal weight gain among adult WIC participants delivering term singleton infants: Variation by maternal and program participation characteristics. *Maternal and Child Health Journal* 3(3):129–140.
Howie, L.D., Parker, J.D., and Schoendorf, K.C.
2003   Excessive maternal weight gain patterns in adolescents. *Journal of the American Dietetic Association* 103(12):1653–1657.
Hytten, F., and Chamberlain, G.
1980   *Clinical Physiology in Obstetrics.* Oxford, Eng.: Blackwell Scientific Publications.
Institute of Medicine
1990   *Nutrition During Pregnancy.* Washington, DC: National Academy Press.
Johnston, C.S., Christopher, F.S., and Kandell, L.A.
1991   Pregnancy weight gain in adolescents and young adults. *Journal of the American College of Nutrition* 10:185–189.
Kopp-Hoolihan, L.E., Van Loan, M.D., Wong, W.W., and King, J.C.
1999   Fat mass deposition during pregnancy using a four-component model. *Journal of Applied Physiology* 87:196–202.
Kouba, S., Hallstrom, T., Lindholm, C., and Hirschberg, A.L.
2005   Pregnancy and neonatal outcomes in women with eating disorders. *Obstetrics and Gynecology* 105(2):255–260.
McFarlane, J., Parker, B., and Soeken, K.
1996   Abuse during pregnancy: Associations with maternal health and infant birth weight. *Nursing Research* 45(1):37–42.
Olafsdottir, A.S., Skuladottier, G.V., Thorsdottir, I., Hauksson, A., and Steingrimsdottir, L.
2006   Maternal diet in early and late pregnancy in relation to weight gain. *International Journal of Obesity* 30(3):492–499.
Olson, C.M., and Strawderman, M.S.
2003   Modifiable behavioral factors in a biopsychosocial model predict inadequate and excessive gestational weight gain. *Journal of the American Dietetic Association* 103(1):48–54.
Scholl, T.O., and Chen, X.
2002   Insulin and the "thrifty" woman: The influence of insulin during pregnancy on gestational weight gain and postpartum weight retention. *Maternal and Child Health Journal* 6:255–261.
Siega-Riz, A.M., and Adair, L.S.
1993   Biological determinants of pregnancy weight gain in a Filipino population. *American Journal of Clinical Nutrition* 57:365–372.
Siega-Riz, A.M., and Hobel, C.J.
1997   Predictors of poor maternal weight gain from baseline anthropometric, psychosocial, and demographic information in a Hispanic population. *Journal of the American Dietetic Association* 97:1264–1268.
Stein, T.P., Scholl, T.O., Schluter, M.D., and Schroeder, C.M.
1998   Plasma leptin influences gestational weight gain and postpartum weight retention. *American Journal of Clinical Nutrition* 68:1236–1240.
Stevens-Simon, C., and McAnarney, E.R.
1992   Determinants of weight gain in pregnant adolescents. *Journal of the American Dietetic Association* 92(11):1348–1351.
Stevens-Simon, C., McAnarney, E.R., and Roghmann, K.J.
1993   Adolescent gestational weight gain and birth weight. *Pediatrics* 92(6):805–809.

Stotland, N.E.
  2006   Gestational Weight Gain: Social Predictors or Relationships. Presentation at the Workshop on the Impact of Pregnancy Weight on Maternal and Child Health, May 30, Washington, DC.
Tok, E., Ertunc, D., Bilgin, O., Erdal, E., Kaplanoglu, M., and Dilek, S.
  2006   PPAR-gamma2 Pro12Ala polymorphism is associated with weight gain in women with gestational diabetes mellitus. *European Journal of Obstetrics Gynecology and Reproductive Biology* May:E-pub.
Wells, C.S., Schwalberg, R., Noonan, G., and Gabor, V.
  2006   Factors influencing inadequate and excessive weight gain in pregnancy: Colorado, 2000–2002. *Maternal and Child Health Journal* 10(1):55–62.
Wolfe, W.S., Sobal, J., Olson, C.M., Frongillo, E.A., and Williamson, D.F.
  1997   Parity-associated weight gain and its modification by sociodemographic and behavioral factors: A prospective analysis in U.S. women. *International Journal of Obesity Related Metabolic Disorders* 21(9):802–810.

4

Maternal Weight, Gestational Weight Gain, and Maternal Health

Weight patterns (underweight and overweight) and gestational weight gain can influence both short- and long-term consequences for maternal health. Understanding the effects of different weight patterns and gestational weight gain on maternal health outcomes requires close examination of the mechanisms that link gestational weight to later health conditions as well as consideration of risk and protective factors that contribute to or inhibit these effects. As discussed in Chapter 3, the relationship between prepregnancy weight and gestational weight gain is complex; their influence on maternal health outcomes is not easily distinguished, and this is reflected in this summary. In light of concerns about rising rates of obesity, the presenters focused their review on the contributions of excessive gestational weight gain and overweight status on maternal health outcomes. This focus is a reflection of the recent research efforts in this area.

SHORT-TERM MATERNAL HEALTH OUTCOMES

Kathleen Rasmussen provided an overview of the consequences of weight gain for women during pregnancy and immediately afterward. Both prepregnancy body mass index (BMI) and gestational weight gain are predictors of maternal health outcomes. These outcomes arise either through direct effects of BMI (prepregnancy or postpartum) or gestational weight gain, or through their interaction. These two factors may operate through the same mechanism, possibly an excess of fat, or through other mechanisms. In general, higher rates of pregnancy weight gain lead to more negative health outcomes; this is particularly true for obese and overweight women. Details of these effects are described below.

Preeclampsia

Preeclampsia is an abnormal state of pregnancy characterized by hypertension and fluid retention and albuminuria; it can lead to eclampsia, preeclampsia combined with seizure-like convulsions, if untreated. A recent study of gestational weight gain and preeclampsia by Cedergren (2006) used data on all births registered in Sweden between 1994 and 2002. The data reflect the country's 96 percent white population. The adjusted odds ratio of developing preeclampsia for women with weight gains of less than 18 lbs. was substantially reduced for all women with a BMI >20 when compared with women who gained between 18 and 35 lbs. Women in all BMI groups who gained more than 35 lbs. were at greater risk of developing preeclampsia than women who gained between 18 and 35 lbs.

Gestational Diabetes Mellitus

Although prepregnant BMI is a well-known predictor of gestational diabetes, the role of gestational weight gain as a separate predictor of this condition has not been demonstrated. An association between total gestational weight gain and diabetes is difficult to interpret, because once a woman is diagnosed with gestational diabetes, her weight gain is often intensely managed. Anna Marie Siega-Riz described a study (Saldana et al., 2005) that examined the relationship between weight gain and glucose intolerance during pregnancy by tracking weight gain up to the time when gestational diabetes was diagnosed. Results showed that the weight gain ratio (observed weight gain over the Institute of Medicine (IOM) recommended weight gain) was higher for women with gestational diabetes when compared statistically with women with normal glucose tolerance. The statistical likelihood of developing gestational diabetes was increased by both prepregnancy overweight and obesity status, while the interaction with weight gain during pregnancy was only marginal. A substantial interaction between prepregnant BMI and gestational weight gain arises when considering impaired glucose tolerance. In this study, women who were classified overweight before pregnancy and who also had excessive gestational weight gain were at a highly increased risk for impaired glucose tolerance when compared with women who had lower gestational weight gain and prepregnancy BMI. In addition, this association was especially strong for black women, suggesting that race/ethnicity may be a moderator of the interaction between prepregnancy BMI and gestational weight gain on glucose intolerance.

Cesarean Delivery

Dietz et al. (2005) used data from the Pregnancy Risk Assessment Monitoring System (PRAMS) to explore the impact of prepregnant BMI and gestational weight gain (independently and in interaction) on cesarean delivery. Statistically, women who were obese or severely obese (BMI >35) before pregnancy had an increased risk of cesarean delivery. In addition, women in the very highest gestational weight gain category (41 lbs. or more) had increased risk of cesarean delivery. There was no interaction between prepregnant BMI and weight gain during pregnancy in this study. In the discussion session, Siega-Riz noted another study with similar results (Vahratian et al., 2005). The possibility of an interaction between pre-pregnancy BMI and gestational weight gain in predicting the likelihood of cesarean delivery was also studied by Cedergren (2006) using a sample of Swedish women. Among women who gained less than 18 lbs. during pregnancy, those who were overweight, obese, or severely obese had a reduced risk of cesarean delivery compared with those who gained 18 to 35 lbs. during pregnancy. And regardless of a woman's prepregnant BMI, gaining more than 35 lbs. compared with gaining 18 to 35 lbs. led to an increased risk of having a cesarean delivery.

Duration of Breastfeeding

Research has suggested an association between prepregnant BMI and failure to initiate and sustain breastfeeding among postpartum women. Inasmuch as the biological mechanism for this association could be the accumulation of fat it is possible that gestational weight gain may also play a role.

Data from PRAMS have not demonstrated an interaction between prepregnant BMI and gestational weight gain on the duration of any breast-feeding, but Rasmussen's recent study of 2,700 women in Cooperstown, New York, reported such an interaction for the duration of exclusive breastfeeding (Hilson et al., 2006). Specifically, gaining more than the IOM recommended weight was associated with shorter breastfeeding duration for underweight women as well as overweight or obese women, when compared with normal-weight women.

Data on U.S. women may reflect the lack of support for breastfeeding in U.S. culture, so it is informative to conduct the same analysis in cultures in which breastfeeding is protected and supported. One such culture is Denmark, where women have 24 weeks of fully paid maternity leave, which encourages longer periods of breastfeeding. Unpublished analyses from 35,000 women in the Danish National Birth Cohort (J.L. Baker and K.M. Rasmussen, unpublished data) provide this counterpoint. In this sample, the risk of early termination of full breastfeeding went up as BMI increased from underweight to normal to overweight to obese. In each BMI group, women who gained the most weight during pregnancy had the highest risk of early termination, and obese women were at risk of early termination of full breastfeeding regardless of how much weight they gained during pregnancy.

Postpartum Weight Retention

To investigate the association between gestational weight gain and postpartum weight retention, Rasmussen compared data from Greene et al. (1988) and from Muscati et al. (1996). Even though the Greene et al. data examined the amount of weight retained between pregnancies (adjusted for the duration between pregnancies) and those of Muscati et al. reported on weight retention at six weeks postpartum, analyses of both datasets suggest the same conclusion; women who gained more than 15.5 lbs. retained weight at the endpoint measured in each data set.

The only data available on minority women and postpartum weight retention are those drawn from the 1988 National Maternal and Infant Health Survey by Keppel and Taffel (1993). In this study, when women's total weight gains were less than the IOM guidelines throughout their pregnancies, retention rates for both black and white women were similar at 10 to 18 months postpartum; the proportion of women who retained more than 14 lbs. was less than 10 percent of white women and about 15 percent of black women. At weight gains within the IOM recommendations, 35 percent of black women retained more than 14 lbs. but only 10 percent of white women did so. At weight gains above the IOM recommendations, proportions of both black and white women retained more than 14 lbs. statistically. Parker and Abrams (1993) have also used this data set to provide information about the gestational weight gain of black women. They found that when compared with white women, black women were consistently more likely to retain 20 lbs. at 10 to 18 months postpartum.

The data from the Bassett Mothers' Health Project allow for a more detailed examination of gestational weight gain and postpartum retention (Olson et al., 2003). In general, in this study heavier women retained more weight if they had gained excessive amounts of weight, although this accounted for relatively little of the variance in postpartum weight retention. In multivariate analysis, Olson et al. demonstrated that a variety of factors predicted postpartum weight retention, including high levels of exercise, low food intake, still breastfeeding at a year postpartum, low gestational weight gain, and extremes of maternal age. One reported statistically significant interaction indicates that lower income women (defined as an annual family income <185 percent of the poverty income ratio) who gained more than the recommended amount of weight were particularly likely to have retained more than 10 lbs. when compared with women with higher incomes. In addition, lower income women who were obese before pregnancy were also likely to retain more weight than obese women with higher incomes.

Finally, data from the Danish National Birth Cohort have been used to examine whether the duration of breastfeeding modifies the relationships between prepregnant BMI, gestational weight gain, and postpartum weight retention (J.L. Baker and the Postpartum Weight Retention Study Group, unpublished, personal communication). In this study, there was a 29 lbs. difference between those who retained the least at 6 months postpartum (obese women who gained below the IOM guidelines and fully breastfed their babies longer than 16 weeks) and those who retained the most (underweight women who gained above the IOM recommendations and breastfed less than 16 weeks). In other words, breastfeeding behavior modified the effects of both prepregnant BMI and gestational weight gain on postpartum weight retention.

Summary of Short-Term Maternal Health Outcomes

Table 4-1 summarizes the information on immediate and short-term maternal outcomes of gestational weight gain and prepregnancy BMI. Rasmussen observed that while more data were available since the 1990 IOM report, understanding these relationships among key variables re-

TABLE 4-1 Presence of an Association for Immediate and Short-Term Maternal Health Outcomes Attributable to Prepregnant Body Mass Index (BMI) and Gestational Weight Gain

Outcome	Prepregnant BMI	Gestational Weight Gain	Interaction
Preeclampsia	Yes	Yes	Unknown
Gestational diabetes	Yes	No	Unknown
Cesarean delivery	Yes	Yes	Conflicting
Failure to initiate/sustain breastfeeding	Yes	Yes	No/conflicting
Postpartum weight retention at 1 year	No	Yes	Conflicting

NOTES: "Yes" indicates an association has been found in the literature between prepregnancy BMI or gestational weight gain to a maternal health outcome. "No" indicates an association has not been found in the literature between prepregnancy BMI or gestational weight gain to a maternal health outcome.
SOURCE: Rasmussen (2006).

mains limited. Information for minority groups is all but unavailable. The available data, however, consistently show associations between increasing prepregnant BMI, more specifically being overweight or underweight, and a range of negative maternal health outcomes—preeclampsia, gestational diabetes, cesarean delivery, failure to initiate and sustain breastfeeding, and postpartum weight retention at 1 year. The data that demonstrate relationships between gestational weight gain and these same negative outcomes are also consistent: excessive weight gain is associated with these same negative maternal health outcomes. What is currently either unknown or inconsistent in the literature is the nature of the interactions between prepregnant BMI (being overweight or underweight) and gestational weight gain in predicting these varied negative maternal health outcomes.

LONG-TERM MATERNAL HEALTH OUTCOMES

Erica Gunderson reviewed current knowledge about long-term health outcomes (more than 1-year postpartum) for mothers as a function of weight gain during pregnancy. In the 1990 IOM report, limited data were available on the effects of gestational weight gain on maternal health; the main concern was how much weight was gained during pregnancy or retained postpartum.

A growing literature on the influence of childbearing on women's health examines not only the first few years after delivery but also subsequent decades. Some of the studies presented and reviewed include a nonpregnancy comparison group, which may help distinguish weight gain due to pregnancy from weight change unrelated to pregnancy. Other studies include only women who have had a pregnancy (pregnancy cohort), which may help identify maternal attributes that contribute to weight gain and retention.

Long-Term Weight Gain

The modifiable attributes or predictors of postpartum weight retention addressed in the 1990 IOM report include prepregnancy weight, parity, gestational weight gain, age, and lactation. Since 1990 a number of additional factors have emerged, which include prepregnancy body size (i.e., BMI), interval to first birth, socioeconomic status, and smoking, as well as the fixed attributes of race/ethnicity and age at menarche (see Table 4-2).

Prepregnancy Weight Patterns

Gunderson explained that researchers and clinicians have been trying to estimate long-term maternal weight gain, which is primarily assessed at

TABLE 4-2 Summary of Attributes of Postpartum Obesity

Before 1990	Since 1990
Modifiable Attributes	Modifiable Attributes
Age	Age
Gestational weight gain	Gestational weight gain
Lactation	Lactation
Prepregnancy weight	Prepregnancy BMI
Parity	Parity
	Internal to first birth
	Socioeconomic status
	Smoking
	Fixed Attributes
	Race/ethnicity
	Age at menarche

SOURCE: Gunderson (2006).

two years after pregnancy, as a function of weight gain during pregnancy. Gunderson indicated that it has been known since 1957 that the heavier a woman is at the beginning of pregnancy (measured by BMI), the greater her weight is later (McKeown and Record, 1957). This weight includes both retained pregnancy gain and weight gained postpartum due to postpartum behaviors. In a Scottish study, overweight women had the greatest increases in body weight before subsequent pregnancies, and most of this was after the first birth (Billewicz, 1970). In other work with a perinatal cohort (Gunderson et al., 2001), higher long-term weight changes for obese women were found despite their lower pregnancy gain, with no real differences observed in BMI groups across race/ethnicity groups.

Recent pregnancy cohort studies, which primarily have included only primiparous women, have looked at long-term excess weight gain after pregnancy. These studies found that at two or more years postpartum, mean weight gain values compared with preconception weight varied somewhat but are estimated generally at about 6 lbs. (McKeown and Record, 1957), about 1.8 lbs. for women who were underweight, and 5.3 lbs. for women who were overweight (Billewicz, 1970). Harris et al. (1997) reported that 71 percent of primiparous women retained less than 2.2 lbs. In a study with women from multiple racial and ethnic groups, weight gain at 2 years postpartum was around 4.4 lbs. for underweight and normal-weight women and about 8.8 lbs. for overweight and obese women (Gunderson et al., 2001). The key risk factors for the excess weight gain after pregnancy, which were fairly consistent across these studies, were high prepregnancy weight, high prepregnancy BMI, high gestational weight gain, and parity.

Pattern of Postpartum Weight Loss

A study from 1957 looked at the pattern of maternal weight loss during the postpartum period by lactation duration (McKeown and Record, 1957). This is one of the few studies that includes serial weight measurements after delivery, in this case three times during the first year and at 24 months postpartum. The study indicates a potential pattern of postpartum maternal weight loss and suggests a point at which there is a change from a loss to a gain.

As mentioned earlier, work done in the pregnancy cohort looked at whether pregnancy gain varied by prepregnancy BMI (Gunderson et al., 2001). The overweight women gained (net gain) the most weight during pregnancy (30 lbs.). What is striking is that the early net postpartum weight change (first 6 weeks) was almost identical across BMI groups, such that early net weight gain did not vary, but late postpartum net weight change varied tremendously (Figure 4-1). In this study, larger declines occurred in the lighter women than the heavier women. From 6 weeks postpartum to a

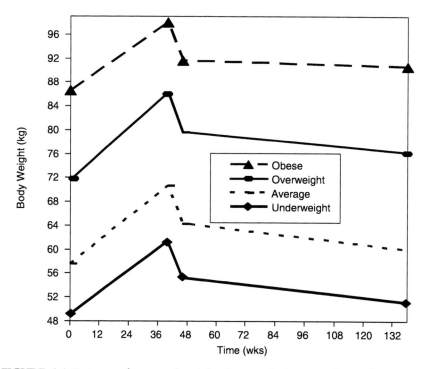

FIGURE 4-1 Patterns of maternal weight changes during gestation and postpartum periods by prepregnancy BMI.
SOURCE: Gunderson et al. (2001). Reprinted by permission from Macmillan Publishers Ltd: *International Journal of Obesity.*

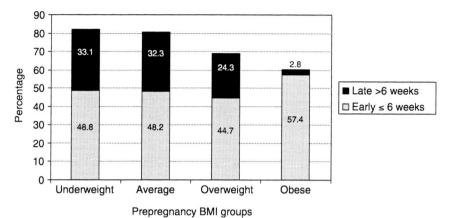

FIGURE 4-2 Net early and late postpartum weight loss as a percentage of net gestational gain by prepregnancy BMI.
SOURCE: Gunderson et al. (2001). Adapted by permission from Macmillan Publishers Ltd: *International Journal of Obesity.*

point 2 years later, there was a downward trend for most of the groups, except for the obese women, whose weight remained steady. After adjusting for secular trends as well as underreporting of preconception weight (because it was between two pregnancies), additional weight gain occurred after 6 weeks postpartum among the obese and the overweight women. Gunderson indicated that as a proportion of the total pregnancy gain, obese women gained the least during pregnancy and 56 percent of their early 6-week weight loss postpartum was due to the pregnancy gain. After 6 weeks, however, their weight loss was a much smaller proportion (only 9 percent), and overall they ended up losing a lower proportion of the pregnancy gain over time compared with women with a prepregnant BMI categorized as underweight, normal, and overweight (Figure 4-2).

Incidence and Correlates of Overweight After Pregnancy

Incidence   Another important outcome that was addressed is the shift in BMI categories. Using 1998 national data, Parker and Abrams (1993) calculated the risk of retaining more than 20 lbs. at 2 years postpartum. Overall, 14 percent of women retained more than 20 lbs. and a higher proportion of black than white women had excessive weight retention. A study of Swedish women indicated that 8 percent became overweight (Ohlin and Rossner, 1994) within a year after pregnancy, and a study of a pregnancy cohort (Gunderson et al., 2000) found that 6.4 percent became overweight within two years after pregnancy. Of those who became overweight, 69 percent had excessive gestational weight gain. A higher proportion of those who became overweight were Hispanics and blacks, and lower proportions were Asians compared with white women.

Correlates   A multivariate model using those same data from the pregnancy cohort looked for associations with excess weight gain postpartum (Gunderson et al., 2001). In this model, excessive gestational weight gain led to a threefold increase in risk of excess weight gain postpartum and a doubling of the risk was associated with increasing age. The researchers also found that women who had short intervals (less than 8 years) between menarche and first birth had a threefold higher risk of excess weight gain postpartum. Age at menarche of less than 12 years, which has been looked at as a predictor of weight change over time, was also independently associated with an almost threefold increase in risk of excess weight gain postpartum. Asian ethnicity was a protective factor for excess weight gain postpartum, with no meaningful increase in risk of excess weight gain postpartum for Hispanics or blacks compared with a white reference group. Gunderson concluded that gestational weight gain is a strong predictor of excess weight gain postpartum, but other biological factors can be strong independent effects.

Gunderson et al. (2004b) and Williamson et al. (1994) have examined childbearing and the risk of becoming overweight. In these studies, they compared women who gave birth to women who did not during a fixed interval. They included preconception measured weights on all the women as well as measured weights during the study follow-up period. Williamson et al. (1994) found that having one birth versus zero doubled the risk of becoming obese. Gunderson et al. (2004b) found an interaction between childbearing and smoking status; for smokers, childbearing reduced the risk of becoming overweight, and for never-smokers childbearing more than doubled the risk of becoming overweight with childbearing (Gunderson et al., 2004b). In addition, in this study, independent of childbearing, black women were 3.5 times more likely to become overweight, whether or not they had a birth (Gunderson et al., 2004b). Parker and Abrams (1993) found overall that women with high gestational weight gain had an increased risk of being overweight postpartum, and this was especially true for black women as compared to white women.

A few studies have looked at whether weight gain during pregnancy might predict weight gain 8 to 15 years later in life (Linne and Rossner, 2003; Rooney and Schauberger, 2002). These studies include only white women and have high attrition rates, but overall their results suggest that high prepregnancy BMI, weight retention at 6 months postpartum, gestational weight gain, and short breastfeeding duration are associated with greater weight gain later in life.

In summary, Gunderson reviewed the incidence and correlates of substantial weight gain after pregnancy (more than 2 years postpartum) based on pregnancy cohort studies. These correlates include high prepregnancy BMI, gestational weight gain greater than the 1990 IOM recommendations, primiparity, short interval from menarche to first birth, and menarche before 12 years of age.

Long-Term Changes in Adiposity

Two prospective studies with data on long-term weight gain for primiparous women and a nonpregnancy comparison group report conflicting results (Coronary Artery Risk Development in Young Adults [CARDIA] and National Health and Nutrition Examination Study [NHANES] Epidemiologic Follow-up Study). The CARDIA study results (a 5- and 10-year study) suggested that primiparous women have excessive weight gain postpartum, about 4 to 7 lbs. more than nulliparous women (who have no births) (Gunderson et al., 2004a; Smith et al., 1994). The NHANES Epidemiologic Follow-up Study (a 10-year study), which involves a smaller number of primiparous women, found that the multiparous women are the ones with excess gain postpartum (Williamson et al., 1994; Wolfe et al., 1997). The CARDIA study (Gunderson et al., 2004a) examined a large sample of women for 10 years and found that, among normal-weight women, the postpartum excess gain due to childbearing was only about 2 lbs. but women who were overweight before pregnancy gained 7 to 13 lbs. This result occurred only among the primiparous women and was the same for blacks and whites. The absolute weight gain among overweight black women was higher than for overweight white women, and the absolute gain in the black normal-weight group was higher than the white normal-weight group. Looking across number of births, the researchers found that among overweight women, black women show 7 to 11 lbs. long-term postpartum weight gain, while white women show an 11 to 13 lbs. gain due to a single birth.

In a follow-up study of the Black Women's Health Survey, the researchers found (over a 4-year period) that primiparous women gained more net weight than nulliparous ones, and excess net weight gain associated with one birth was about 7 lbs. for overweight women, who also had some increase in BMI with gestational weight gain (Rosenberg et al., 2003). An increase in BMI was found among women who gained more than 25 lbs. during pregnancy.

Other Long-Term Health Outcomes

Independent of weight gain, other conditions associated with childbearing—such as abdominal obesity, plasma lipid changes, and an increased risk of chronic disease, including coronary heart disease and diabetes—may affect women's health.

Abdominal Obesity

The CARDIA study measured waist girth to gain insight into the association between childbearing and abdominal obesity (Gunderson et al., 2004a; Smith et al., 1994). Waist girth was measured in this prospective study at preconception for those who bore children and these women were compared with a nongravid (not pregnant) reference group. Primiparous women gained more abdominal girth than nulliparous women (Gunderson et al., 2004a; Smith et al., 1994). There is a similar association with excess gains in waist circumference for normal-weight and overweight women (primiparous and multiparous). Normal-weight women (both black and white) showed about 1 inch excess waist girth gain, and overweight black and white women showed very similar excess gain of 1.5 and 2.5 inches, respectively (Gunderson et al., 2004a).

Plasma Lipid Changes

There also appears to be an association between higher parity and with lower high-density lipoprotein (good cholesterol) levels, and in cross-sectional studies, researchers have found a threshold effect with a high number of births. However, in the best prospective studies of women of childbearing age, having one birth (versus none) contributed to a drop of 3.5 mg/dl on average (Lewis et al., 1996). In the longer term (10 years), there appears to be a 3 to 4 mg/dl difference between primiparous and nulliparous women, with similar changes for black and white women (Gunderson et al., 2004a).

Chronic Diseases

In terms of pregnancy and future risk of chronic disease, a study using a pregnancy cohort found that a high BMI and excess weight gain over 15 years were associated with increased risk of future chronic disease although the researchers did not report a direct association between gestational weight gain and chronic disease (Rooney et al., 2005). Higher lifetime parity has been associated with coronary heart disease risk in women, but the data are conflicting (Colditz et al., 1987; Ness et al., 1994; Rosenberg et al., 1999; Steenland et al., 1996). Diabetes has also been associated with lifetime parity in several early studies, but this association was confounded by age, fertility, socioeconomic status, and BMI.[1]

---

[1]Although not presented at the workshop, it is important to note that other health outcomes may exist in relation to maternal weight and gestational weight gain.

Cross-sectional and population-based studies of the association of parity with type II diabetes have produced conflicting results. A single prospective study reported no association between parity and diabetes when age, BMI, and family history of diabetes were controlled (Manson et al., 1992). For women with gestational diabetes, there is some evidence that an additional pregnancy is associated with a threefold higher risk of type II diabetes, independent of weight gain (Peters et al., 1996).

Research Needs

The workshop discussion sessions identified many gaps in the existing body of knowledge. First, understanding the influence of social determinants of health on maternal weight is a major priority. Second, studies should explore the risk of chronic disease (type II diabetes, hypertension, arthritis, cancers) by prepregnancy weight or gestational weight gain and the impact of these factors on not only weight but also abdominal adiposity, body composition, and other risk factors for cardiovascular disease. Third, the field needs more information about preconception measures of the risk factors, gestational weight gain, postpartum weight patterns, whether postpartum weight gain is really retention or secular trends, and what point in time is the most important to intervene. Fourth, research is needed that examines lactation and long-term weight changes in women. Finally, there are few data on Hispanic or Asian women.

Summary of Long-Term Maternal Health Outcomes

In summary, cumulative gains in abdominal obesity, lower high-density lipoprotein levels independent of obesity, and weight gain during midlife are all associated with increased risk of chronic diseases in women. There is some evidence about an increased risk of diabetes after experiencing gestational diabetes. However, the evidence is insufficient about whether childbearing itself is associated with these chronic diseases, or whether the gain over time is due to factors other than childbearing.

The greatest long-term health effects of childbearing (>1-year postpartum) appear to occur after a first birth. These effects occur mostly among women who were already overweight before pregnancy and who have excessive weight gain after pregnancy, higher waist girth, and lower high-density lipoprotein values. Among normal-weight women, there is a modest increase in the risk of postpartum overweight following childbirth as well as a cumulative effect with each birth on waist girth. The long-term health effects of childbearing do not seem to differ by race/ethnicity as long as maternal obesity at the start of pregnancy is taken into account.

SUMMARY

At the workshop, Rasmussen and Gunderson reviewed research on maternal health outcomes of gestational weight gain. Understanding the effects of different weight patterns (overweight or underweight) and gestational weight gain on maternal health outcomes requires further attention to a broad array of factors associated with the status of women's health in different demographic groups. New data exist on the consequences of insufficient or excessive gestational weight gain for women, but these data are limited in scope. Recent research efforts focus more on being overweight and excessive gestational weight gain as risk factors for poor maternal health outcomes. Information for minority groups primarily includes only non-Hispanic black U.S. women; almost no data are available on Hispanic, Asian, or Native American populations of women.

Although limited, the data available consistently show associations between prepregnant BMI and a range of negative immediate and short-term maternal health outcomes (<1-year postpartum) including preeclampsia, gestational diabetes, cesarean delivery, failure to initiate and sustain breast-feeding, and postpartum weight retention at 1 year. Studies that show a relationship between gestational weight gain and these same immediate and short-term maternal health outcomes are also consistent. However, whether or not there is an interaction between prepregnant BMI (overweight or underweight) and gestational weight gain in predicting immediate and short-term maternal health outcomes is unknown or inconsistent in the literature.

A limited yet growing literature has demonstrated the influence of childbearing on women's long-term maternal health outcomes (>1-year postpartum). This research base generally uses (1) prospective studies, which may help distinguish weight gain due to pregnancy from weight change unrelated to pregnancy, and (2) pregnancy cohort studies, which may help identify maternal attributes that contribute to weight gain and retention. This body of research has suggested that cumulative gains in abdominal obesity, lower high-density lipoprotein levels independent of the obesity, and weight gain during midlife are all associated with increased risk of chronic diseases in women. However, the evidence is insufficient about whether the childbearing experience is associated with these chronic diseases specifically, or whether the gain over time is due to factors other than childbearing. More research is needed on the impact of childbearing independent from and in combination with additional risk factors on long-term health outcomes. There is some evidence suggesting an increased risk of diabetes after experiencing gestational diabetes. The most serious longer term maternal health outcomes of childbearing appear to occur mostly among women who were already overweight before pregnancy, have excessive gains in weight and waist girth after pregnancy, and have lower high-density lipoprotein levels. In addition, among women with a normal BMI there is a modest increase in the risk of overweight postpartum, and each birth has a cumulative effect on waist girth.

The high rates of obesity among women of reproductive age suggest that guidelines that are directed solely at changing gestational weight gain should be viewed as only one component of a comprehensive strategy to limit the long-term maternal effects of chronic obesity. Since the ability to predict gestational weight gain is limited and the consequences of inappropriate gestational weight gain are poorly understood, more research is necessary to inform the knowledge base that could guide policy and professional guidance. At a minimum, attention needs to focus on prepregnancy weight status and gestational weight gain, independently and in combination, as strong indicators of subsequent weight gain trends. Additional attention needs to be paid to the adolescent population, since the nature and strength of these relationships may differ from those found among older mothers.

REFERENCES

Billewicz, W.Z.
   1970   Body weight in parous women. *British Journal of Preventive Social Medicine* 24(2): 97–104.
Cedergren, M.
   2006   Effects of gestational weight gain and body mass index on obstetric outcome in Sweden. *International Journal of Gynaecology and Obstetrics* 93(3):269–274.
Colditz, G.A., Willett, W.C., Stampfer, M.J., Rosner, B., Speizer, F.E., and Hennekens, C.H.
   1987   A prospective study of age at menarche, parity, age at first birth, and coronary heart disease in women. *American Journal of Epidemiology* 126(5):861–870.
Dietz, P.M., Callaghan, W.M., Morrow, B., and Cogswell, M.E.
   2005   Population-based assessment of the risk of primary cesarean delivery due to excess prepregnancy weight among nulliparous women delivering term infants. *Maternal and Child Health Journal* 9(3):237–244.
Greene, G.W., Smiciklas-Wright, H., Scholl, T.O., and Karp, R.J.
   1988   Postpartum weight change: How much of the weight gained in pregnancy will be lost after delivery? *Obstetrics and Gynecology* 71(5):701–707.
Gunderson, E.P.
   2006   Childbearing, Gestational Gain and Long-term Effects on Women's Health: Obesity and Chronic Disease. Presentation at the Workshop on the Impact of Pregnancy Weight on Maternal and Child Health, May 30, Washington, DC.
Gunderson, E.P., Abrams, B., and Selvin, S.
   2000   The relative importance of gestational gain and maternal characteristics associated with the risk of becoming overweight after pregnancy. *International Journal of Obesity Related Metabolic Disorders* 24(12):1660–1668.
   2001   Does the pattern of postpartum weight change differ according to pregravid body size? *International Journal of Obesity Related Metabolic Disorders* 25(6):853–862.

Gunderson, E.P., Murtaugh, M.A., Lewis, C.E., Quesenberry, C.P., West, D.S., and Sidney S.
  2004a   Excess gains in weight and waist circumference associated with childbearing: The Coronary Artery Risk Development in Young Adults study (CARDIA). *International Journal of Obesity Related Metabolic Disease* 28(4):525–535.
Gunderson, E.P., Quesenberry, C.P., Lewis, C.E., Tsai, A.L., Sternfeld, B., West, D.S., and Signey, S.
  2004b   Development of overweight associated with childbearing depends on smoking habit: The Coronary Artery Risk Development in Young Adults (CARDIA) study. *Obesity Research* 12(12):2041–2053.
Harris, H.E., Ellison, G.T., Holliday, M., and Lucassen, E.
  1996   The impact of pregnancy on the long-term weight gain of primiparous women in England. *International Journal of Obesity and Metabolic Disorders* 21(9):747–755.
Hilson, J.A., Rasmussen, K.M., and Kjolhede, C.L.
  2005   Excessive weight gain during pregnancy is associated with earlier termination of breast-feeding among white women. *Journal of Nutrition* 136(1):140–146.
Institute of Medicine
  1990   *Nutrition During Pregnancy.* Washington, DC: National Academy Press.
Keppel, K.G., and Taffel, S.M.
  1993   Pregnancy-related weight gain and retention: Implications of the 1990 Institute of Medicine guidelines. *American Journal of Public Health* 83(8):1100–1103.
Lewis, C.E., Funkhouser, E., Raczynski, J.M., Signey, S., Bild, D.E., and Howard, B.V.
  1996   Adverse effect of pregnancy on high density lipoprotein (HDL) cholesterol in young adult women. The CARDIA study: Coronary Artery Risk Development in Young Adults. *American Journal of Epidemiology* 144(3):247–254.
Linne, Y., and Rossner, S.
  2003   Interrelationships between weight development and weight retention in subsequent pregnancies: The SPAWN study. *Acta Obstetrics et Gynecology Scandanavia* 82(4): 318–325.
Manson, J.E., Rimm, E.B., Colditz, G.A., Stampfer, M.J., Willett, W.C., Arky, R.A., Rosner, B., Hennekens, C.H., and Speizer, F.E.
  1992   Parity and incidence of non-insulin-dependent diabetes mellitus. *American Journal of Medicine* 93(1):13–18.
McKeown, T., and Record, R.G.
  1957   The influence of weight and height on weight changes associated with pregnancy in women. *Journal of Endocrinology* 15:423–429.
Muscati, S.K., Gray-Donald, K., and Koski, K.G.
  1996   Timing of weight gain during pregnancy: Promoting fetal growth and minimizing maternal weight retention. *International Journal of Obesity Related Metabolic Diseases* 20(6):526–532.
Ness, R.B., Schotland, H.M., Flegal, K.M., and Shofer, F.S.
  1994   Reproductive history and coronary heart disease risk in women. *Epidemiological Reviews* 16(2):298–314.
Ohlin, A., and Rossner, S.
  1994   Trends in eating patterns, physical activity and socio-demographic factors in relation to postpartum body weight development. *British Journal of Nutrition* 71(4): 457–470.
Olson, C.M., Strawderman, M.S., Hinton, P.S., and Pearson, T.A.
  2003   Gestational weight gain and postpartum behaviors associated with weight change from early pregnancy to 1 yr postpartum. *International Journal of Obesity Related Metabolic Disorders* 27(1):117–127.

Parker, J.D., and Abrams, B.
  1993   Differences in postpartum weight retention between black and white mothers. *Obstetrics and Gynecology* 81(5 Pt 1):768–774.
Peters, R.K., Kjos, S.L., Xiang, A., and Buchanan, T.A.
  1996   Long-term diabetogenic effect of single pregnancy in women with previous gestational diabetes mellitus. *Lancet* 347(8996):227–230.
Rasmussen, K.M.
  2006   Gestational Weight Gain: Short-term Maternal Health Outcomes. Presentation at the Workshop on the Impact of Pregnancy Weight on Maternal and Child Health, May 30, Washington, DC.
Rooney, B.L., and Schauberger, C.W.
  2002   Excess pregnancy weight gain and long-term obesity: One decade later. *Obstetrics and Gynecology* 100(2):245–252.
Rooney, B.L., Schauberger, C.W., and Mathiason, M.A.
  2005   Impact of perinatal weight change on long-term obesity and obesity-related illnesses. *Obstetrics and Gynecology* 106(6):1349–1356.
Rosenberg, L., Palmer, J.R., Rao, R.S., and Adams-Campbell, L.L.
  1999   Risk factors for coronary heart disease in African American women. *American Journal of Epidemiology* 150(9):904–909.
Rosenberg, L., Palmer, J.R., Wise, L.A., Horton, N.J., Kumanyika, S.K., and Adams-Campbell, L.L.
  2003   A prospective study of the effect of childbearing on weight gain in African-American women. *Obesity Research* 11(12):1526–1535.
Saldana, T.M., Siega-Riz, A.M., Adair, L.S., and Suchindran, C.
  2005   The relationship between pregnancy weight gain and glucose tolerance status among black and white women in central North Carolina. *American Journal of Obstetrics and Gynecology* July 3: E-pub.
Smith, D.E., Lewis, C.E., Caveny, J.L., Perkins, L.L., Burke, G.L., and Bild, D.E.
  1994   Longitudinal changes in adiposity associated with pregnancy. *Journal of the American Medical Association* 271(22):1747–1751.
Steenland, K., Lally, C., and Thun, M.
  1996   Parity and coronary heart disease among women in the American Cancer Society CPS II population. *Epidemiology* 7(6):641–643.
Vahratian, A., Siega-Riz, A.M., Savitz, D.A., and Zhang, J.
  2005   Maternal pre-pregnancy overweight and obesity and the risk of primary cesarean delivery in nulliparous women. *Annals of Epidemiology* 15(7):467–474.
Williamson, D.F., Madams, J., Pamuk, E., Flegal, K.M., Kendrick, J.S., and Serdula M.K.
  1994   A prospective study of childbearing and 10-year weight gain in U.S. white women 25 to 45 years of age. *International Journal of Obesity Related Metabolic Disorders* 18(8):561–569.
Wolfe, W.S., Sobal, J., Olson, C.M., Frongillo, E.A., and Williamson, D.F.
  1997   Parity-associated weight gain and its modification by sociodemographic and behavioral factors: A prospective analysis in U.S. women. *International Journal of Obesity Related Metabolic Disorders* 21(9):802–810.

5

Maternal Weight, Gestational Weight Gain, and Children's Health

A major session of the workshop addressed the role of maternal weight and gestational weight gain as direct predictors and moderators of children's growth and health. Matthew Gillman introduced the session by observing that the 1990 Institute of Medicine (IOM) report placed an emphasis on birth outcomes that are chiefly related to low birth weight, which was a particular concern at that time. However, in this current era of epidemic obesity, attention has expanded the range of birth weight outcomes of interest as well as other salient short- and long-term outcomes for which birth weight is a proxy. Gillman also discussed fetal and developmental origins of chronic disease, and the life-course approach, which postulates that perturbations during the earliest stages of human development can have lifelong impact on chronic disease. Gillman expressed the view that the human development model may be an important key in understanding the effects of maternal weight and weight patterns during pregnancy on infants' and children's growth and health.

The following sections review the available research on short-term infant health outcomes and the long-term child health outcomes of maternal and gestational weight gain. In general, short-term health outcomes refer to infants up to 1 year of age. Long-term health outcomes refer to children over 1 year. Although the charge to the committee is a focus on infant health outcomes (up to 12 months), several presenters also reviewed literature on older child health outcomes of maternal and gestational weight gain, and this research is reflected in this chapter. The primary focus of this review is the influence of excessive gestational weight gain and overweight pregnancies on child health outcomes, reflecting recent research trends.

SHORT-TERM INFANT HEALTH OUTCOMES

Patrick Catalano provided an overview of the impact of prepregnancy maternal weight and gestational weight gain on the fetus. Specifically, he discussed preterm delivery, intrauterine growth restriction, macrosomia, and body composition. As mentioned in Chapter 2, statistical increases have occurred in prepregnancy weight in women of childbearing age. The prevalence of obesity has nearly doubled from the 1980s to early 2000, to close to 30 percent. In addition, data from MetroHealth Medical Center in Cleveland show the mean maternal weight at the time of delivery has increased to 190 lbs. in 2003, up from 170 lbs. in 1987.

Preterm Delivery

Maternal prepregnancy weight and gestational weight gain are related to preterm delivery.[1] A recent meta-analysis of 13 studies published from 1980 through 1996 concluded that inadequate weight gain is associated with an increased risk of prematurity, with a possible indication specifically on inadequate gain late in pregnancy (Carmichael and Abrams, 1997). Overall, about 75 percent of preterm deliveries are not medically indicated but occur from spontaneous labor due to premature rupture of the membranes. In the past 10 years, an increased number of multiple births has also occurred, which are frequently associated with preterm deliveries. Approximately one-quarter of all preterm births are indicated on the basis of maternal complications, such as hypertension, diabetes, and preeclampsia. Women at the greatest risk for having a preterm birth are those with a history of preterm birth, with about three to four times the baseline population risk.

Analyses using the Pregnancy Nutrition Surveillance System show that the risk of preterm delivery varied by both maternal prepregnancy body mass index (BMI) and gestational weight gain (Schieve et al., 1999). The lowest risk of preterm delivery was found in women gaining between 0.6 and 1 lb per week, and the highest preterm delivery rate was to women who gained below or above these parameters. The greatest risk was to those women with a low prepregnancy BMI and a gestational weight gain of less than 0.2 lb/week. Similar results were found using the National Maternal

---

[1]Many other factors relate to preterm delivery. More information can be found in the IOM report *Preterm Birth: Causes, Consequences, and Prevention* (Institute of Medicine, 2007).

and Infant Health Survey excluding medically indicated preterm deliveries (Schieve et al., 2000), and analyzing data from the Pregnancy Risk Assessment Monitoring System (Dietz et al., 2006).

Preterm risk associations with gestational weight gain may be related to maternal adipose tissue and cytokine production, because preterm delivery is related to a maternal or fetal inflammatory response. In addition, recent studies indicate that inadequate gestational weight gain and low prepregnancy BMI are associated with an increased risk of premature deliveries; the highest risk was found in underweight women who gained little weight during pregnancy. Although a substantial increase in BMI has occurred in women of reproductive age, the preterm delivery rates in the United States have steadily increased in the past 20 years from about 8 to about 12 percent (Mercer et al., 2006). This trend suggests that other factors are influencing preterm birth in addition to prepregnancy BMI and gestational weight gain, especially since an increase in prepregnancy BMI should be protective against preterm birth.

Mercer conducted a secondary analysis of the preterm prediction study, a component of the Maternal Fetal Medicine Network Units of the National Institute on Child Health and Human Development, looking at factors related to preterm delivery (Mercer et al., 2006). He compared four groups: (1) women who had recurrent term births only (two or three term births), (2) women with no history of any preterms, (3) women who had an isolated spontaneous preterm birth and a term birth in between, and (4) women who were at the highest risk of recurrent spontaneous preterm births, with two or three spontaneous preterm births and no interval term pregnancy. He further divided women who had isolated spontaneous preterm births based on whether this delivery was prior to or was itself the index pregnancy for the study. Results showed that 38 percent of women with low prepregnancy BMI (less than 19.8) and recurrent spontaneous preterm births delivered preterm. Compared with women with either recurrent term births or isolated spontaneous preterm births, those women with a low prepregnancy BMI had a greater risk of another spontaneous preterm delivery. The women who had recurrent spontaneous preterm births had a greater risk of low BMI and low weight gain in the early part of pregnancy. The women who had the recurrent spontaneous preterm births also had the shortest cervixes compared with the other groups, a characteristic related to their BMI, not to their height. Levels of maternal plasma cytokines, in this particular instance IL-6, were lower in the women who had recurrent spontaneous preterm births; women who were lean and had recurrent spontaneous preterm births had lower values. In conclusion, women with recurrent spontaneous preterm births weigh less and are leaner before and during the pregnancy, have shorter cervixes and an advanced Bishop score (an indication of readiness to induce birth) by 22 to 24 weeks related to the prepregnancy weight but not their height, and they deliver at an earlier gestational age than those who did not have an isolated spontaneous preterm birth in their current pregnancy.

Intrauterine Growth Restriction

Maternal prepregnancy weight and gestational weight gain are also related to intrauterine growth restriction. Most people define intrauterine growth restriction as less than 10 percent weight for gestational age, adjusting for gender, race, and geography, primarily altitude. Many different factors contribute to intrauterine growth restriction, including fetal placental factors, such as chromosomes, genetic syndromes, congenital malformations, infectious disease, and placental pathologies. Other factors include such medical problems as maternal hypertension, diabetes, particularly involving vasculopathies, low maternal prepregnancy weight, premature labor, hypoxia, and substance abuse.

Catalano stated that poor maternal weight gain in pregnancy has not been found to be directly related to the risk of intrauterine growth restriction.[2] For example, in the Dutch winter famine of 1945, women in the latter part of pregnancy were severely restricted in their calories, but the average birth weight decreased by only 240 grams. In data published in 2002, the number of term small-for-gestational-age births that occurred from 1985 through 1998 decreased in both the white and the black populations by 11 to 12 percent in the United States; in Canada, the numbers decreased by 27 percent (Ananth and Wen, 2002).

Macrosomia

On the other extreme are babies born with extremely high birth weights, or macrosomia, defined as birth weight greater than 90th percentile, and also referred to as large for gestational age. A commonly used criterion is 4,000 grams (about 9 lbs.), but this confounds some of the important predictors of macrosomia, notably gestational age, the most important factor, as well as altitude, socioeconomic status, and race/ethnicity. International data suggest an increasing incidence of macrosomic births. In Denmark in the past 10 years the mean birth weight has increased 45 grams, and the number of babies greater than 9 lbs. has increased to 20 percent (Orskou et al., 2001). In Sweden during the same time period there has

---

[2]It is important to note that in *Nutrition During Pregnancy*, the IOM reported a positive relationship of gestational weight gain on gestational age-adjusted birth weight and the risk of intrauterine growth restriction (Institute of Medicine, 1990).

been a 23 percent increase in the incidence of large babies, which is related to an increase in maternal BMI and a decrease in smoking (Surkan et al., 2004). The incidence of term babies large for gestational age has increased between 5 and 9 percent in the United States during the same time period, and in Canada up to 24 percent (Ananth and Wen, 2002). The epidemiological data show the number of large-for-gestational-age babies seems to be increasing in the population.

Finally, Catalano looked at data from Cleveland's MetroHealth Medical Center dating back to 1975, which shows a mean increase in birth weight of 116 grams. The rate of birth of large babies, variously defined, is increasing, a trend that is primarily related to maternal prepregnancy weight.

Infant Body Composition

Catalano examined an emerging area of research on body composition at birth in humans and its possible relationship to maternal weight and gestational weight gain. Humans, of all the mammalian species, have the greatest amount of body fat at the time of delivery, around 12 to 15 percent. Studies have considered lean body mass to have a genetic component, and fat mass may be reflecting the intrauterine environment (Sparks, 1984).

One study of women with normal glucose tolerance and women with gestational diabetes looked at the factors relating to fetal growth as indexed by body composition measures (see Box 5-1) (Catalano and Ehrenberg, 2006). Attributable variance of the infant's birth weight, lean body mass, fat mass, and percentage body fat were calculated. Gestational age is the strongest predictor of infant birth weight, followed by maternal prepregnancy weight, maternal gestational weight gain, smoking (as a negative factor), and parity. These factors account for 24 percent of the total variance in birth weight. Infant lean body mass at birth was predicted by gestational age (the strongest predictor), smoking, maternal prepregnancy weight and maternal weight gain during pregnancy, parity, maternal height, and genetic influence. These factors account for a total of about 25 percent of the variance. Maternal prepregnancy BMI has the strongest correlation with infant fat mass at the time of delivery (among term singleton infants). Gestational age is an important predictor of infant fat mass, but maternal gestational weight gain accounts for only about half of the variance of infant fat mass compared with variance accounted for by maternal prepregnancy BMI. Even though close to half of the women had gestational diabetes with a known risk factor for macrosomia, it accounted for only about 1.6 percent of the variance of about 19 percent explained. The data for percentage body fat were similar to fat mass for the infant, maternal

---

BOX 5-1

**Major Maternal Factors That Relate to Fetal Growth and
Body Composition in Infants in a Population of Women
with Gestational Diabetes and Women with
Normal Glucose Tolerance**

Birth Weight
  Gestational age
  Prepregnancy weight
  Weight gain
  Smoking (–)
  Parity

Lean Body Mass
  Gestational age
  Smoking (–)
  Prepregnancy weight
  Weight gain
  Parity
  Maternal height
  Paternal weight

Fat Mass
  Prepregnancy BMI
  Gestational age
  Weight gain
  Gestational diabetes

% Body Fat
  Prepregnancy BMI
  Gestational age
  Weight gain
  Gestational diabetes

NOTE: Listed in order of attributable variance (most variance, to least variance).
SOURCE: Catalano and Ehrenberg (2006). Reprinted with the permission of the Royal College of Obstetricians and Gynaecologists.

---

prepregnancy BMI being the strongest correlate, gestational age followed by maternal weight gain during pregnancy, and gestational diabetes.

One study compared the body composition of neonates born to lean normal-weight women (prepregnancy BMI less than 25) and women who were overweight or obese (BMI greater than or equal to 25) prior to their pregnancy (Sewell et al., 2006). In this one study, infant birth weight was slightly greater (not statistically significant) for the prepregnancy overweight and obese women compared with the lean normal-weight women. Among other body composition variables, there was no difference in infant lean body mass between the two groups of mothers. However, the women who were overweight or obese before pregnancy had infants who had a greater the amount of fat mass and percentage body fat than the lean normal-weight women. Prepregnancy BMI was not predictive of infant lean body mass, but gestational age was the best predictor of infant lean body mass in women who were lean and of average weight before pregnancy. Percentage body fat for the infant was predicted by gestational age plus the fetal gender (female) for the lean average weight. Considering the women who were overweight or obese before they got pregnant, gestational age plus fetal gender (male) correlated with infant lean body mass. In women who were overweight or obese prior to pregnancy, maternal weight gain in pregnancy, the 1-hour glucose screen, and gestational age contributed to the infant's percent body fat.

Summary of the Short-Term Infant Health Outcomes

The review by Catalano at the workshop indicated that lower rates of maternal prepregnancy weight and gestational weight gain increase the risk of preterm delivery.[3] There has been a substantial increase in infant birth weight concomitant with the increase in maternal weight over the past decade. Gestational age is the strongest predictor of fetal fat mass. In addition, fetal fat mass has a stronger correlation with maternal prepregnancy BMI than gestational weight gain. Finally, for women who are overweight and obese prior to conception, an increase in maternal weight gain during pregnancy is correlated with an increase in fetal adiposity.

LONG-TERM CHILD HEALTH OUTCOMES

Emily Oken presented an overview of the literature on longer term (>1 year) health outcomes for children based on maternal weight and weight gain during pregnancy. Child weight patterns (based on BMI) are the primary outcome of interest in this literature. Limited information is available about fat and lean body proportions in offspring or about the central distribution of body fat, which is predictive of disease risk. Just a handful of studies have looked at cardiovascular risk factors, including blood pressure, lipids, glucose intolerance, and insulin resistance, as well as type II diabetes and cardiovascular disease. Finally although higher weight at birth has been linked with increased risk for cancer, such as breast cancer in particular, and lower weight at birth is associated with increased risk for osteoporosis and schizophrenia, the existing literature does not link these conditions to maternal weight. Therefore, a number of intermediate steps occur in the pathway linking maternal weight and gestational weight gain to child health outcomes.

This section reviews what is known about the effect of maternal weight and weight gain during pregnancy on child health outcomes.

---

[3]Although not presented at the workshop, it is important to note that additional infant health outcomes may relate to maternal weight and gestational weight gain.

Early Life Factors and Other Considerations

Several factors may influence the association of maternal weight and weight gain during pregnancy with long-term child health outcomes. These include glucose tolerance during pregnancy, birth weight, fetal growth, smoking during pregnancy, infant feeding practices, and maternal and paternal BMI.

Higher maternal weight is a risk factor for gestational diabetes or glucose tolerance during pregnancy, as noted in Chapter 4. A fairly robust body of evidence now suggests that children born to mothers who had diabetes during pregnancy are themselves at higher risk for overweight, gestational diabetes, and type II diabetes. These risks appear to be independent of the maternal prepregnancy weight.

As discussed in the previous section, many studies have demonstrated a direct association between birth weight and higher BMI in childhood and adulthood. There is also an extensive body of evidence suggesting an association between lower fetal growth and increased risk for obesity, glucose intolerance, and cardiovascular disease risk, even after adjusting for offspring BMI. Finally, more rapid growth in the first months, and even perhaps the first days of postnatal life, are associated with increased risk for child overweight.

Maternal and paternal BMI reflect the shared genes in the environment between parents and child, so adjusting for parental size is important for isolating the role of the prenatal environment. Paternal weight data have generally not been as readily available as maternal weight data. When present, paternal weight tends to be less strongly linked with child weight, which may suggest a persistent influence of the intrauterine environment. Oken and others have shown that smoking during pregnancy is associated with increased risk for child overweight.

Mothers who gain more weight and who are more overweight may be less likely to breastfeed, and breastfeeding protects against later child obesity. Overweight mothers may also be more likely to introduce solid foods earlier, and early introduction of solids is also a risk factor for later development of obesity.

The pathways linking maternal weight and weight gain with child outcomes are somewhat complex (Figure 5-1). It is important to consider the extent to which maternal weight and weight gain during pregnancy act independent of these pathways, because they may help to clarify the population impact of greater pregnancy obesity and higher gestational weight gains.

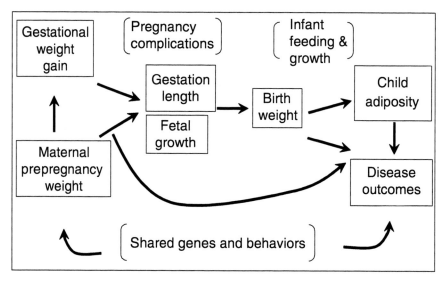

FIGURE 5-1 Relationship of maternal weight and pregnancy weight gain to child outcomes.
SOURCE: Oken (2006).

Maternal Weight

In a study of low-income children in the Special Supplemental Food Program for Women, Infants, and Children (WIC), Whitaker (2004) found a linear association between maternal BMI (in the first trimester) and the odds of overweight in 2-, 3-, and 4-year-old children. A second study in Denmark found a direct association between maternal BMI and offspring BMI and also reported the strengthening of this association with increasing offspring age into adulthood (Schack-Nielsen et al., 2005).

A study of men and women in China suggests that, after adjustment for offspring BMI, lower maternal BMI was associated with increased glucose, increased insulin, and increased low-density lipoprotein (bad cholesterol) levels in the offspring (Mi et al., 2000). It is important to note that, in this study, maternal BMI was measured at 15 weeks gestation and is low compared with current U.S. BMI levels.

A study of about 3,000 adult men with data from birth in Finland found an indirect association between size at birth and cardiovascular disease mortality (Forsen et al., 1997). Offspring of mothers who had higher BMI at the end of their pregnancies were at elevated risk for cardiovascular disease. This association was limited to mothers who were below average height in the population. The authors conclude that since height is an indicator of early life nutrition, a mother who was undernourished in early life but then became overnourished in later life confers elevated cardiovascular disease risk for her offspring. However, these risks were not adjusted for offspring BMI, so it is not clear whether they were mediated through higher obesity in the offspring or an independent association of maternal BMI on child cardiovascular disease risk.

In summary, a linear relationship exists between maternal weight and child weight. This relationship is in part mediated through fetal growth, may become stronger with increasing offspring age, and certainly reflects shared genes and behaviors between mother and child but also perhaps demonstrates a persistent effect of the fetal intrauterine environment. There is limited information about child health outcomes other than weight in relation to maternal weight.

Gestational Weight Gain

Very few published studies examine gestational weight gain and child outcomes. Studies that have included gestational weight gain use it as a covariate but not as a primary predictor, so it is not clear that interactions and associations were completely explored.

Fisch et al. (1975) suggest an association between gestational weight gain and child weight. Data from the Collaborative Perinatal Project showed that mothers of babies who were above the 95th percentile (weight for height) at birth had a higher mean gestational weight gain than mothers of babies who were below the 5th percentile (weight for height) at birth. These associations persisted into childhood, although they were less strong and no longer statistically significant (not adjusted for maternal weight, birth weight, or any other factors). Another study, using data from a different subpopulation of the Collaborative Perinatal Project, reported that the association of gestational weight gain with child weight was null (Stettler et al., 2000).

The Danish cohort study discussed earlier reported a linear association of maternal gestational weight gain with offspring BMI that appears to be fairly consistent across ages (Schack-Nielsen et al., 2005). It is also associated with child gender, fetal growth, maternal age, sociodemographics and smoking. The authors report that they saw no interaction between maternal prepregnancy BMI and gestational weight gain. In a larger study of Israelis who were born in the 1970s, Seidman et al. (1996) indicated higher gestational weight gain was associated with an elevated odds ratio of offspring overweight. A study of over 1,000 children in Italy born in the 1970s and early 1980s found no association between gestational weight gain and child weight, although gestational weight gain was assessed retrospectively and by recall only (Maffeis et al., 1994). This is the only study to show an inverse association of gestational weight gain with BMI and percentage body fat.

A more recent study by Whitaker (2004) with a large population of children enrolled in the WIC program shows no obvious linear association of gestational weight gain with child overweight risk, and in fact suggests a J shape with a higher risk in the first quartile, lower in the second, and then perhaps increasing. Gestational weight gain here was obtained from birth certificates and was reported as net weight gain, not total weight gain, and was adjusted for maternal but not paternal BMI, smoking, sociodemo-graphics, and fetal growth. The authors reported no interaction between BMI and gestational weight gain.

Oken described initial data analyzed from Project Viva, a long-term pregnancy and child cohort study with information on over 1,000 children, followed to age 3. In the study, maternal and child weight are very similar to current national estimates. These data suggest a linear association be-tween maternal gestational weight gain and the risk of child overweight at age 3, child BMI score, and the sum of subscapular and triceps skinfolds. There was no association between gestational weight gain and the ratio of subscapular to triceps skinfolds, which is a measure of central obesity. Increased gestational weight gain was also associated with increase of sys-tolic blood pressure, adjusted for maternal prepregnancy BMI, smoking, race/ethnicity, income, marital status, glucose tolerance during pregnancy, paternal BMI, child gender, gestation length, and breastfeeding duration. Final adjustment estimates remain statistically meaningful, suggesting that gestational weight gain has an independent effect on child overweight and child BMI at age 3. Looking at maternal weight gain (using IOM catego-ries), compared with mothers who gained inadequate weight, mothers who gained both adequate and excessive weight had similar elevations in the child's BMI score.

Finally, Oken described one study that suggests the relationship be-tween maternal gestational weight gain and child overweight risk seems to vary within different categories of maternal prepregnancy weight; it as-sumes a J shape among underweight mothers, a U shape among mothers with gestational weight gain less than 45 lbs., and a linear pattern at the highest weight gains (personal communication, A.J. Sharma, Centers for Disease Control and Prevention). The lowest risk of child overweight was seen in mothers who were underweight before pregnancy and gained less than 45 lbs. and the highest absolute risk of overweight was seen in mothers who were obese before pregnancy and gained 30 lbs. or more.

Research Needs

Potential areas for future research include studies to examine cohorts using the recommended IOM prepregnancy BMI categories and gestational weight gain, measures of body fat distribution and disease risk as well as just BMI, and longer follow-up of infants born in this current era of obesity. One way of overcoming the limitations of the observational studies would be to follow children whose mothers were enrolled in trials targeting gestational weight gain, to see whether those children whose mothers receive interventions to reduce their gestational weight gain have lower attained weight. Nearly all of the data presented here are from developed populations, with no real presence of nutritionally compromised populations and few minorities. Finally, there is little direct information about mechanisms by which weight and weight gain might influence offspring weight, although it is possible to extrapolate from studies of gestational diabetes and also from animal studies. Some animal models that might be informative include experimental induction of gestational diabetes in rats, injection of insulin or glucocorticoids into the pregnant mother to examine effects on offspring, and neonatal overfeeding of rats.

Summary of Long-Term Infant and Child Health Outcomes

In summary, Oken's review of the literature suggests a direct association of maternal weight and gestational weight gain with offspring overweight, but some exceptions to these findings deserve notice. The associations seem to be in part mediated through fetal growth. The shape of the association varies among women with differing profiles of prepregnancy weight and gestational weight gain, so it is not entirely clear, and not many studies have sufficient data to look at the broad range of gestational weight gain. The interaction between maternal BMI and gestational weight gain is not consistent across published studies. However, many of these data come from previous generations with different prevalence of obesity and gestational weight gain; many were not adjusted for important potential covariates and pathway variables, and all of them are observational studies.

SUMMARY

In summary, maternal BMI and gestational weight gain are higher than in the past. These trends are associated with the increasing prevalence of macrosomia (large-for-gestational-age) infants as well as decreasing rates of small-for-gestational-age infants. Low prepregnancy BMI and inadequate gestational weight gain, in combination, are associated with preterm birth, but maternal BMI is also independently related. A few studies describe the relationship of gestational weight gain and infant body composition. Maternal BMI and gestational weight gain have been shown to predict fat mass and percentage fat in newborns and maternal BMI and gestational weight gain can also predict infant lean body mass. It is unknown what body composition in the newborn predicts for the child weight composition in the long term. It is also unknown if maternal fat gain, not just gestational weight gain, predicts child health outcomes.

In long-term child outcomes, the literature suggests that both BMI and gestational weight gain independently predict risk of overweight in children. There are limited data on obesity-related physiological or morbid outcomes, such as metabolic and cardiovascular risk factors.

Research is limited on body composition, which is difficult to measure in a clinical setting. In addition, the role of the placenta may give insight into the complex mechanism and relationship between maternal weight and child health outcomes. In studying complex interactions among maternal weight, gestational weight gain, and infant and child health outcomes, investigations need to use statistical models that build on conceptual theories. There is a compelling need to examine these relationships in a more diverse population.[4]

Finally, these findings need to be interpreted and referenced through the application of a theoretical model that can lend both coherence and additional research. A life-course approach to chronic diseases offers important promise. This intervention framework includes prenatal, postnatal, biological, environmental, and behavioral characteristics that may occur at many dynamic stages of the mother's and her child's lives. It also incorporates different causal models, including the critical (or sensitive period) model, as well as an accumulation of risk model. In addition, investigations need to consider the relative merits of a public health approach compared with individualized approaches in addressing weight gain and body composition before, during, and after pregnancy.

REFERENCES

Ananth, C.V., and Wen, S.W.
　　2002　Trends in fetal growth among singleton gestations in the United States and Canada, 1985 through 1998. *Seminars in Perinatology* 26(4):260–267.
Carmichael, S.L., and Abrams, B.
　　1997　A critical review of the relationship between gestational weight gain and preterm delivery. *Obstetrics and Gynecology* 89(5 Part 2):865–873.
Catalano, P., and Ehrenberg, H.
　　2006　The short- and long-term implications of maternal obesity on the mother and her offspring. *BJOG: An International Journal of Obstetrics and Gynecology* July 7: E-pub DOI: 10.1111/j.1471-0528.2006.00989.x.
Dietz, P.M., Callaghan, W.M., Cogswell, M.E., Morrow, B., Ferre, C., and Schieve, L.A.
　　2006　Combined effects of prepregnancy body mass index and weight gain during pregnancy on the risk of preterm delivery. *Epidemiology* 17:170–177.

---

[4]Although not presented at the workshop, it is important to note that additional factors may affect infant and child health outcomes.

Fisch, R.O., Bilek, M.K., and Ulstrom, R.
 1975   Obesity and leanness at birth and their relationship to body habits in later child-
        hood. *Pediatrics* 56(4):521–528.
Forsen, T., Eriksson, J.G., Tuomilehto, J., Teramo, K., Osmond, C., and Barker, D.J.
 1997   Mother's weight in pregnancy and coronary heart disease in a cohort of Finnish
        men: Follow up study. *British Medical Journal* 315(7112):837–840.
Institute of Medicine
 1990   *Nutrition During Pregnancy.* Washington, DC: National Academy Press.
 2007   *Preterm Birth: Causes, Consequences, and Prevention.* Washington, DC: The Na-
        tional Academies Press.
Maffeis, C., Micciolo, R., Must, A., Zaffanello, M., and Pinelli, L.
 1994   Parental and perinatal factors associated with childhood obesity in north-east Italy.
        International Journal of Obesity Related Metabolic Disorders 18(5):301–305.
Mercer, B.M., Macpherson, C.A., Goldenberg, R.L., Goepfert, A.R., Haugel-De Mouzon, S.,
Varner, M.W., Iams, J.D., Meis, P.J., Moawad, A.H., Miodovnik, M., Caritis, S.N., Van
Dorsten, J.P., Sorokin, Y., Thurnau, G.R., and Spong, C.Y.
 2006   Are women with recurrent spontaneous preterm births different from those with-
        out such history? *American Journal of Obstetrics and Gynecology* 194(4):1176–
        1184.
Mi, J., Law, C., Zhang, K.L., Osmond, C., Stein, C., and Barker, D.
 2000   Effects of infant birthweight and maternal body mass index in pregnancy on com-
        ponents of the insulin resistance syndrome in China. *Annals of Internal Medicine*
        132(4):253–260.
Oken, E.
 2006   Maternal Weight and Gestational Weight Gain as Predictors of Long-Term Off-
        spring Growth and Health. Presentation at the Workshop on the Impact of Preg-
        nancy Weight on Maternal and Child Health, May 30, Washington, DC.
Orskou, J., Kesmodel, U., Henriksen, T.B., and Secher, N.J.
 2001   An increasing proportion of infants weight more than 4000 grams at birth. *Acta
        Obstetrics and Gynecology Scandanavia* 80(10):931–936.
Schack-Nielsen, L., Mortensen, E.L., and Sorensen, T.I.A.
 2005   High maternal pregnancy weight gain is associated with an increased risk of obesity
        in childhood adulthood independent of maternal BMI. *Pediatric Research* 58(5):
        1020.
Schieve, L.A., Cogswell, M.E., and Scanlon, K.S.
 1999   Maternal weight gain and preterm delivery: Differential effects by body mass in-
        dex. *Epidemiology* 10(2):141–147.
Schieve, L.A., Cogswell, M.E., Scanlon, K.S., Perry, G., Ferre, C., Blackmore-Prince, C., Yu,
S.M., and Rosenberg, D.
 2000   Prepregnancy body mass index and pregnancy weight gain: Associations with pre-
        term delivery. The NMIHS Collaborative Study Group. *Obstetrics and Gynecology*
        96(2):194–200.
Seidman, D.S., Laor, A., Shemer, J., Gale, R., and Stevensen, D.K.
 1996   Excessive maternal weight gain during pregnancy and being overweight at 17 years
        of age. *Pediatric Research* 39:112A.
Sewell, M.F., Huston-Presley, L., Super, D.M., and Catalano, P.
 2006   Increased neonatal fat mass, not lean body mass, is associated with maternal obe-
        sity. *American Journal of Obstetrics and Gynecology* 195(4):1100–1103.
Sparks, J.W.
 1984   Human intrauterine growth and nutrient accretion. *Seminars in Perinatology* 8(2):
        74–93.

Stettler, N., Tershakovec, A.M., Zemel, B.S., Leonard, M.B., Boston, R.C., Katz, S.H., and Stallings, V.A.
   2000   Early risk factors for increased adiposity: A cohort study of African American subjects followed from birth to young adulthood. *American Journal of Clinical Nutrition* 72(2):378–383.
Surkan, P.J., Hsieh, C.C., Johansson, A.L., Dickman, P.W., and Cnattingius, S.
   2004   Reasons for increasing trends in large for gestational age births. *Obstetrics and Gynecology* 104(4):720–726.
Whitaker, R.C.
   2004   Predicting preschooler obesity at birth: The role of maternal obesity in early pregnancy. *Pediatrics* 114(1):e29–e36.

6

Promoting Appropriate Maternal Weight During and After Pregnancy

Workshop participants focused explicitly on insights from interventions to promote appropriate maternal weight during pregnancy and postpartum. Such interventions include individual approaches to change behaviors related to appropriate weight, psychosocial factors that affect weight, community approaches to promote weight management, and practices and policies for clinicians and health systems. The presenters focused their review on interventions to control excessive gestational weight gain. This focus is a reflection of the recent research efforts in this area. In addition to the presentations on determinants of gestational weight gain summarized in Chapter 3, the approaches described in this chapter may help guide Title V maternal and child health programs to assist women of childbearing age to achieve and maintain recommended weight before, during, and after pregnancy.

INDIVIDUAL APPROACHES

Rena Wing presented an overview of strategies to encourage appropriate weight gain during pregnancy. The key times for intervention efforts are during pregnancy, to prevent excessive weight gain during pregnancy, and the postpartum period.

Researchers and practitioners know a great deal about weight management: in order to change their weight, people need to change their energy balance through a combination of caloric restriction and physical activity. Physical activity, although very important for the maintenance of weight loss, actually has a smaller impact on actual production of weight loss. In studies looking at the role of physical activity alone or in combination with diet, physical activity is responsible for only a 2 to 4 lbs. weight change. To lose weight, many individuals need help to change their behaviors, by using such techniques as goal-setting, receiving feedback on the changes, self-monitoring or writing down information, stimulus control (changing the environment they live in), and problem solving. Merely educating individuals about how much to eat and how much to exercise is not sufficient.

Energy Balance Behavior Studies

During Pregnancy

Olson and Strawderman (2003) surveyed 458 pregnant women and asked about changes in their diet and exercise behaviors during their pregnancy. This prospective cohort study followed women from early pregnancy until two years postpartum. Of these women, 41 percent exceeded the 1990 Institute of Medicine (IOM) recommendations for weight gain. Individuals who reported eating much more food during pregnancy than before had a more than twofold risk of exceeding the weight recommendations, and those who reported less physical activity than before pregnancy had a 1.75 relative risk of exceeding the IOM recommendations.

In the study of Icelandic women by Olafsdottir et al. (2006), 34 percent of the women exceeded the IOM recommendations. One of the strongest predictors of doing so was their self-reported caloric intake; women who exceeded IOM recommendations reported consuming 2,186 calories per day, about 300 calories more per day than those with optimal gestational weight gain. This study also reported that increased intake of sugar and fat was related to increased risk of excessive gestational weight gain.

Postpartum

Several studies found that caloric intake and caloric expenditure are related to postpartum weight retention. In Olson and Strawderman's data (2003), 25 percent of the women retained 10 lbs. or more. Individuals who reported increasing food intake during the second 6 months had a more than threefold risk of greater weight retention at the end of the year, and those who reported exercising often actually had a decreased risk of high postpartum weight retention. These studies suggest that the key behaviors to focus on both during pregnancy and afterward are eating and physical activity behaviors that have an impact on energy balance.

Intervention Studies

During Pregnancy

Polley et al. (2002) conducted a randomized control trial to prevent excessive gestational weight gain with 120 women with low-risk pregnancies. The women were enrolled at less than 20 weeks gestation, with body mass index (BMI) greater than 19.8. The control group received the usual care during their pregnancy, while the intervention group received written and oral information about appropriate gestational weight gain, exercise, and healthy eating during pregnancy. They received biweekly newsletters emphasizing these three messages. Both the control and intervention groups include black (39 percent) and non-Hispanic white (61 percent) women who were considered of normal weight (54 percent) or overweight or obese (46 percent). All women in the intervention received goal-setting assistance and feedback. If women continued to exceed the gestational weight gain goal, they received either face-to-face counseling at their clinic visits or phone-based counseling. They also received increasingly structured behavioral goals, both for physical activity and for diet. The study was statistically effective for the normal-weight women; in the control group, 58 percent of the women exceeded the IOM recommendations versus 33 percent in the intervention group. In the overweight group, there was no statistically significant difference.

This intervention during pregnancy showed effectiveness at preventing excessive weight gain in normal-weight women. There was a strong correlation between weight gain during pregnancy and weight retention 1-year postpartum in normal-weight women, arguing for interventions during the pregnancy period to prevent weight retention 1-year postpartum.

There are advantages and disadvantages to intervening during pregnancy. One major advantage of intervening at this time is that excessive weight gain during pregnancy is one of the strongest predictors of subsequent obesity and problems with postpartum weight retention. The major disadvantage to intervening at this time involves psychological concerns about the mother as well as concerns about the developing baby. Interventions to control weight during pregnancy must avoid any potential for harm to the fetus.

Postpartum

Another strategy is to intervene in the postpartum period, allowing the woman to gain what she wants and then dealing with it later. Leermakers et al. (1998) performed a small study of reducing postpartum weight retention. The researchers developed a correspondence intervention targeted at women (97 percent non-Hispanic white) who had delivered within the past 3 to 7 months and who were exceeding their prepregnancy weight by 15 lbs. with a BMI greater than 22 (on average they were exceeding by 27 lbs.).

The women were randomly assigned to a 6-month behavioral treatment through correspondence or a no-treatment control. The correspondence program began with two face-to-face group meetings and continued with 16 weeks of correspondence intervention: behavioral lessons were sent to the women, they completed homework, and they received telephone contact to reinforce progress. The women also followed a 1,000 to 1,500 calorie/day diet. They were encouraged to be physically active and to increase their activity by walking two miles a day five days a week. The no-treatment control group received only informational brochures.

On average the women in the correspondence group lost 17 lbs. over the 6 months compared with 10 lbs. in the control group, a statistically significant difference. About a third of the women in the intervention group returned to their prepregnancy weight, compared with about 11 percent of the controls.

Intervening during the postpartum period can be intensive and involve strict diet and more physical activity. This is an advantage that interventions during pregnancy do not have. There are generally fewer concerns about safety, especially for the child. A disadvantage of postpartum interventions is that it is clearly a burden for new mothers; there was a 31 percent attrition rate in the Leermakers et al. (1998) study. In another study of postpartum weight retention interventions (e.g., O'Toole et al., 2003), only 23 of the 40 women finished the program.

Summary of Individual Approaches

Wing observed that opportunities for interventions exist before pregnancy, during pregnancy, and postpartum, although the literature reviewed included only interventions during pregnancy and postpartum. Setting goals for weight, eating, and activity in addition to feedback for meeting these goals are key components of this type of intervention. Exercise alone and changing the quality of the diet alone do not show an effect of weight loss postpartum.

PSYCHOSOCIAL APPROACHES

Lorraine Walker presented research on psychosocial factors that could affect appropriate weight during pregnancy and postpartum. According to Kramer et al. (2000), psychosocial variables may be mediators of psychosocial disparities in a society, and they may also be antecedents of pathways for changes in physical activity and diet. Although many psychosocial factors may play a role in gestational weight gain, four seem especially important: stress, social support, depression, and attitude. Another factor, infant feeding practices (reviewed in Chapter 4), includes duration of breastfeeding and postpartum weight retention. The literature in these areas is predominantly observational research, often exploratory, rather than theory- or hypothesis-driven.

Psychosocial Factors During Pregnancy

Stress

High stress can have an adverse effect on gestational weight gain, either through behavioral pathways that often are not fully specified or biological pathways leading to inadequate or excessive gestational weight gain. The relationship between stress and BMI is curvilinear, not linear. The literature suggests that stress has different kinds of effects depending on a person's response, an effect also seen with respect to depression. For stress in relation to gestational weight gain, the findings are mixed; different subgroups had positive, negative, or no effects. A few studies indicated that stress was associated with lower gestational weight gain (Brawarsky et al., 2005; Campbell et al., 1999; DiPietro et al., 2003; Hickey et al., 1995; Johnson et al., 2002; Orr et al., 1996; Parker et al., 1994; Picone et al., 1982; Siega-Riz and Hobel, 1997; Stevens-Simon and McAnarney, 1992, 1994; Wells et al., 2006). Stress in these studies includes stressful life events, chronic stress, hassles, or perceived stress in addition to physical or sexual abuse during pregnancy. The lack of consensus on the stress measures challenges comparability of the studies.

Social Support

Social support is typically seen as having a beneficial effect, although the behavioral or biological pathways are not clearly articulated. Social support may have a buffering effect, in that it may cancel the effects of stress on gestational weight gain. However, studies on social support show mixed results, depending on the analysis (DiPietro et al., 2003; Hickey et al., 1995; Olson and Strawderman, 2003; Siega-Riz and Hobel, 1997; Stevens-Simon and McAnarney, 1992). Social support was measured in a variety of ways, including total support, partner support, emotional support, financial support, and network size. None of these studies looked at the possible interaction of social support and stress, although an early study done by Nuckolls et al. (1972) found that women with high stress and low social support had less favorable pregnancy outcomes.

Depression

Maternal depression is usually assessed by an interview administered by a health professional using diagnostic criteria. Most epidemiological studies use a questionnaire that has a cutoff score, such as the Edinburgh Postnatal Depression Scale or the Center for Epidemiologic Studies Depression Scale. Depression is hypothesized to have an adverse effect on gestational weight gain through behavioral or biological pathways, which may lead either to inadequate or excessive gestational weight gain.

About half of the studies looking at a relationship between depression and pregnancy outcomes reported no effect; the remainder indicated mixed effects for subgroups or different associations between high and low gestational weight gain (Brawarsky et al., 2005; DiPietro et al., 2003; Hickey et al., 1995; Siega-Riz and Hobel, 1997; Stevens-Simon and McAnarnery, 1992; Walker and Kim, 2002; Zuckerman et al., 1989). None of the studies looked at the curvilinear relationship between depression and gestational weight gain.

Attitudes

Attitudes are another factor that has been studied in relation to gestational weight gain. Attitudes may relate to either an increase or a decrease in health-promoting or health risk behaviors and may lead to excessive or inadequate gestational weight gain. These factors include attitudes toward pregnancy or weight gain during pregnancy, self-efficacy, motherhood, and career. The results of these studies on attitudes affecting gestational weight gain are mixed; the effects may be seen in one subgroup but not in another (Copper et al., 1995; DiPietro et al., 2003; Olson and Strawderman, 2003; Palmer et al., 1985; Stevens-Simon et al., 1993). One study found that more positive attitudes were related to higher gestational weight gain, but further testing on a more diverse sample showed that negative attitudes toward gestational weight gain were related to more weight gain as well. A critical shortcoming in this area is measurement.

Potential Sources of Information

Data available in some state service models (e.g., California, Colorado) are potential sources of information on the efficacy of psychosocial interventions on promoting appropriate gestational weight gain (Ricketts et al., 2005; Zimmer-Gembeck and Helfand, 1996). In these models, the researchers examined whether or not someone has actually received a psychosocial intervention, whether or not that psychosocial problem has been resolved, and the outcome. Many of those studies may not have gestational weight gain as one of their outcomes.

Psychosocial Factors and Postpartum Weight Retention

The relationship of psychosocial factors and postpartum weight retention was studied. Studies on psychosocial factors and postpartum weight retention are limited to exploratory (rather than theory-driven), primarily observational, studies. Four studies have addressed the area of stress, social support, depression, and their relationship to postpartum weight retention (Walker, 1996, 1997; Walker and Freeland-Graves, 1998; Walker et al., 2004). The studies found no support for the relationship between stress and a high retained weight postpartum. There was some evidence of a relationship between social support and a decrease in retained weight postpartum. The data were split (one study finding a relationship of high retained weight and one finding no effect) regarding the relationship of depressive symptoms and retained weight. In addition, four studies have addressed the effect of attitudes on postpartum weight retention (Walker, 1996; Walker and Grobe, 1999; Walker and Freeland-Graves, 1998; Walker et al., 2004). The attitude variables included weight-related distress (an attitude of dissatisfaction toward one's body image), the pros and cons of weight loss, and the locus of control. Looking at these studies, locus of control was unrelated to postpartum weight retention, and weight-related distress was positively related to a higher gestational weight gain.

Summary of Psychosocial Approaches

Although the evidence on how psychosocial factors relate to weight both during pregnancy and postpartum is inconsistent, the impact of psychosocial factors may be underestimated because of measurement and data analytic issues. Future research could provide a better foundation for examining psychosocial factors, with model-driven tests of the impact of psychosocial factors on gestational weight gain and postpartum weight retention, which could build in some of the behavioral components.

COMMUNITY APPROACHES

Christine Olson presented data from a few studies on the effects of community or multilevel interventions to promote appropriate weight during pregnancy and postpartum. Peterson et al. (2002) describe important features of community interventions addressing multiple levels of influence on diet, physical activity, and weight loss in postpartum women. Their design included a sustained, multiple-component intervention with home visits by a mentor, who targets awareness of weight issues and nutrition, motivation, skill building, and building social support; group classes that reinforce the project messages by teaching and demonstrating some skills as well as fostering social interactions; and telephone counseling. Only two studies are available to provide insight into the effects of these interventions.[1]

Intervention Studies

The first published community intervention study (Gray-Donald et al., 2000) focused on reducing weight gain in pregnancy as a way to prevent gestational diabetes in indigenous communities in Canada. This prospective study, with an 8-month control period followed by a 9-month intervention period, was implemented in four Cree communities in Quebec. The intervention was offered by nutritionists and native health workers. Its design was based on social learning theory and included modeling of the behavior change, skill training, contracting, and self-monitoring. The types of activities the investigators carried out in the community include radio broadcasts, information pamphlets, supermarket tours and cooking demonstrations, exercise walking groups, and individualized nutrition counseling.

The study results indicated no statistically significant differences between the control and intervention groups in such outcomes as weight gain during pregnancy, plasma glucose, and weight and weight retention at 6 weeks postpartum. The results of this study could be confounded with cultural norms of Cree communities; physical activity is not considered appropriate during pregnancy, and being plump is normal.

The second intervention study, Staying in the Range, sought to decrease weight retention at 1-year postpartum by promoting appropriate gestational weight gain in a health care system in Cooperstown, New York (Olson et al., 2004). The goal was to decrease (by 50 percent) the proportion of normal and overweight BMI women who exceeded the upper limit of the 1990 IOM gestational weight gain recommendations (Institute of Medicine, 1990). This prospective cohort study included a historical control group from an observational study with usual care in pregnancy and an intervention group. The intervention group was followed from early pregnancy through a postpartum period with measures of gestational weight gain and weight retained at 1-year postpartum. The design of the intervention included health care providers monitoring weight gain using adapted IOM gestational weight gain grids. The pregnant women received five motivational action-promoting newsletters and postcards focusing on their gestational weight gain, diet, and physical activity, and they also received a

---

[1]Although not presented at the workshop, it is important to note that some promising techniques and tools are emerging that offer potential components for future evidence-based intervention studies.

health checkbook for goal-setting and self-monitoring. The process evaluation indicated most women engaged with the postcards, setting appropriate gestational weight gain goals.

Based on the data collected, the intervention had a statistically significant effect on decreasing excessive gestational weight gain in the low-income women only. A three-way interaction among income, treatment, and BMI was found on postpartum weight retention. In addition, reduced weight retention was seen at 1-year postpartum for the overweight low-income women.

HEALTH SYSTEM APPROACHES

Laura Riley highlighted factors of health care and of the health care system that could promote or hinder the compliance of recommended gestational weight guidelines prior to, during, and after pregnancy. There is scant literature on this topic. Riley focused on the recommended practices and policies that are available for clinicians in promoting appropriate weight prior to, during, and after pregnancy. She closed her presentation with personal clinical experiences.

Guidelines

American College of Obstetrics and Gynecology Guidelines

The American College of Obstetrics and Gynecology (ACOG) issues short committee reports with specific recommendations as well as the underlying science and data. Reports from the OB Practice Group and the GYN Practice Group give guidelines on addressing obesity in pregnancy for obstetricians, gynecologists, and other health professionals or paraprofessionals, and highlight the role of the obstetrician and gynecologist in the assessment and management of obesity.

The OB Practice Group (American College of Obstetricians and Gynecologists, 2005) presented a strong argument that obstetricians should provide preconception counseling and education about the complications that may be faced by obese patients and encourage these patients to undertake a weight reduction program before attempting pregnancy. Suggestions include recording patients' height and weight; offering nutrition counseling; and screening for gestational diabetes earlier in pregnancy than the standard 28 weeks gestation.

Other parts of the ACOG guidelines include anesthesia consultation, which is important for obese women, who have higher rates of cesarean delivery and other complications. The report also includes discussion on antibiotic prophylaxis; postoperative complications specific to the obese population; and fetal monitoring challenges. Finally, since more women are having bariatric surgery prior to pregnancy, ACOG guides obstetricians on the differences in their pregnancies.

Another ACOG report, issued by the GYN Practice Group, is equally important for the topic of this workshop. The GYN Practice Group issued guidelines on the assessment and management of obesity in nonpregnant women, which is important to clinicians who provide preconception care (American College of Obstetricians and Gynecologists Committee on Gynecologic Practice, 2005). It stresses calculating BMI and then offering overweight patients appropriate interventions or referrals to promote healthy weight and lifestyle. The report also provided information about patients who may benefit from pharmacotherapy or for whom a consultation about surgery should be considered.

Another ACOG committee on adolescent health care has decided to review issues specific to overweight adolescents. They are pulling together data concerning prevention, treatment, and obstetric as well as gynecological implications. This will provide preconception information for young women as well as for those who experience unintended pregnancies.

The *Guidelines for Perinatal Care* (5th edition) addresses some of the issues with obesity and includes the IOM recommendations for weight gain during pregnancy (American Academy of Pediatrics and American College of Obstetricians and Gynecologists, 2002). The 6th edition will include an expanded discussion about appropriate weight gain and the potential implications of obesity in pregnancy. *Guidelines for Women's Health Care* (2nd edition) includes a discussion about weight gain, healthy lifestyle, and healthy eating (American College of Obstetricians and Gynecologists, 2002).

Guidelines from Other Groups

Other professional organizations are providing similar guidance. The American Academy for Family Physicians does not have specific documents similar to the ACOG committee reports; however, its web site provides information for members about screening and advises physicians to screen all adult patients for obesity and to offer intensive counseling and behavioral interventions to promote sustained weight loss for obese adults.

The American College of Midwives expresses interest in the topic. Although they do not currently have resources to produce their own document, they encourage the use of the IOM recommendations and reprint them in various places. They have conducted two major educational series that included the topic of obesity through lectures at their annual meetings, one of which was published in their journal.

Evaluation of Guidelines

Do these professional efforts make a difference in terms of how providers treat their patients? ACOG administered a survey to a random sample of practitioners one year before its committee reports were issued (prior to 2004) to test practitioner knowledge about obesity, as well as to determine practice patterns before the committee reports were released. A second, one-year postcommittee opinion survey has been distributed, but data are not yet available.

The Massachusetts General Hospital Experience

Following the OB Practice Group's report on obesity in pregnancy, Riley investigated the obstetrician patient population of Massachusetts General Hospital. Although the ACOG reports target individual practice, large health care systems can also change their practice based on these guidelines. A preliminary review of 3,500 obstetric patients through electronic medical records revealed that 40 percent of the patient population was overweight or obese at the time of their first prenatal visit. Hispanic and black women had the highest rates of obesity and overweight. A total of 54 percent of the population was overweight or had obesity at their postpartum visit, which is generally 6 to 8 weeks postpartum. About 25 percent of women gained more than 35 lbs. during their pregnancy.

All providers received a paper about the impact of obesity on health that focused on pregnancy and issues surrounding childbirth, including both maternal and fetal complications. This information was most helpful to the nurses, who do a fair amount of patient education. Massachusetts General is planning to conduct focus groups to learn more about obesity and pregnancy. They want to understand the relevance to the clinicians' practice, how to understand the patients' perception of the problem, what interventions would work best in each particular group, and how to support patients as well as clinicians.

From a practice perspective, a number of practical considerations arise in moving toward implementation of the ACOG recommendations. Concerns include availability and cost of nutrition counseling; the number of obese women who will seek preconception counseling; and payment for preconception counseling. The practice pattern of internal medicine physicians concerning preconception counseling for obese women needs to be understood. Finally, there is a need for more research on the effectiveness of intervention efforts for this specific population.

SUMMARY

Interventions to promote appropriate weight during pregnancy and postpartum include individual (behavior), psychosocial, community, and health care and health care system approaches. Studies on the design or impact of interventions delivered before pregnancy to promote appropriate weight gain during pregnancy are not available. The presenters focused their review on interventions to control excessive gestational weight gain, consistent with recent research efforts in this area.

Individual approaches to change behavior are based on achieving an energy balance between diet and physical exercise. Studies have focused on interventions to limit excess weight gain during pregnancy and weight retention in the postpartum period. Behavioral strategies include goal-setting, feedback, self-monitoring, stimulus control, and problem solving. Psychosocial factors may affect appropriate weight during pregnancy and postpartum as well. These factors include stress, social support, depression, attitudes, and infant feeding practices. The studies that investigate the effect of these factors on pregnancy-related weight are inconsistent in their findings; all are observational studies with methodological problems that make it difficult to interpret them.

A community-based intervention is based on a multilevel sustained approach to promote appropriate gestational weight gain and reduce postpartum weight retention. The study design can include home visits, social support, group classes, goal-setting, skill training, self-monitoring, and feedback. Compared with individualized approaches, community-based programs may be a less expensive approach with low clinician burden. Finally, no studies exist on clinician or health care and health care system–based interventions to improve pregnancy-related weight gain. Practice guidelines available for obstetricians and gynecologists include assessment and management of obesity and pregnancy, as well as interventions for women with a history of bariatric surgery. However, the guidelines are not likely to be implemented in isolation; evidence on the effectiveness of behavioral interventions suggests that behavioral modification components will be necessary to add to the guidelines so that health providers can offer more comprehensive or additional support to women during prepregnancy and perinatal periods.

It is important that approaches to achieve and maintain recommended weight before, during, after, and between pregnancies are investigated. The appropriate approach may vary by subgroup. Studies on interactions of variables, prepregnancy BMI and gestational weight gain, race/ethnicity and gestational weight gain, and socioeconomic status and gestational weight gain are needed. A combination of these approaches, at the individual and the environmental levels, may be required for women to achieve and maintain recommended weight before, during, and after pregnancy. Indeed, integration of weight management into a healthy lifestyle is a critical goal.

In addition to these approaches (individual, psychosocial, community, and clinician and health system), the presentations on determinants of gestational weight gain in Chapter 3 offer insight for Title V maternal and child health programs to help women of childbearing age to achieve and maintain recommended weight before, during, and after pregnancy.

REFERENCES

American Academy of Pediatrics and American College of Obstetricians and Gynecologists
  2002   *Guidelines for Perinatal Care.* 5th ed. Elk Grove Village, IL: American Academy of Pediatrics and American College of Obstetricians and Gynecologists.
American College of Obstetricians and Gynecologists
  2002   *Guidelines for Women's Health Care.* 2nd ed. Washington, DC: American College of Obstetricians and Gynecologists.
  2005   ACOG committee opinion number 315, September 2005. Obesity in pregnancy. *Obstetrics and Gynecology* 106(3):671–675.
American College of Obstetricians and Gynecologists Committee on Gynecologic Practice
  2005   ACOG committee opinion number 319, October 2005. The role of obstetrician-gynecologist in the assessment and management of obesity. *Obstetrics and Gynecology* 106(4):895–899.
Brawarsky, P., Stotland, N.E., Jackson, R.A., Fuentes-Afflick, E., Escobar, G.J., Rubashkin, N., and Haas, J.S.
  2005   Pre-pregnancy and pregnancy-related factors and the risk of excessive or inadequate gestational weight gain. *International Journal of Gynaecology and Obstetrics* 91(2):125–131.
Campbell, J., Torres, S., Ryan, J., King, C., Campbell, D.W., Stallings, R.Y., and Fuchs, S.C.
  1999   Physical and nonphysical partner abuse and other risk factors for low birth weight among full term and preterm babies: A multiethnic case-control study. *American Journal of Epidemiology* 150(7):714–726.
Copper, R.L., DuBard, M.B., Goldenberg, R.L., and Oweis, A.I.
  1995   The relationship of maternal attitude toward weight gain to weight gain during pregnancy and low birth weight. *Obstetrics and Gynecology* 85(4):590–595.
DiPietro, J.A., Millet, S., Costigan, K.A., Gurewitsch, E., and Caulfield, L.E.
  2003   Psychosocial influences on weight gain attitudes and behaviors during pregnancy. *Journal of the American Dietetic Association* 103(10):1314–1319.
Gray-Donald, K., Robinson, E., Collier, A., David, K., Renaud, L., and Rodrigues, S.
  2000   Intervening to reduce weight gain in pregnancy and gestational diabetes mellitus in Cree communities: An evaluation. *Canadian Medical Association Journal* 163(10): 1247–1251.
Hickey, C.A., Cliver, S.P., Goldenberg, R.L., McNeal, S.F., and Hoffman, H.J.
  1995   Relationship of psychosocial status to low prenatal weight gain among nonobese black and white women delivering at term. *Obstetrics and Gynecology* 86(2):177–183.
Institute of Medicine
  1990   *Nutrition During Pregnancy.* Washington, DC: National Academy Press.

Johnson, P.J., Hellerstedt, W.L., and Pirie, P.L.
  2002   Abuse history and nonoptimal prenatal weight gain. *Public Health Reports* 117(2):
          148–156.
Kramer, M.S., Seguin, L., Lydon, J., and Goulet, L.
  2000   Socioeconomic disparities in pregnancy outcome: Why do the poor fare so poorly?
          Paediatric and Perinatal Epidemiology 14(3):194–210.
Leermakers, E.A., Anglin, K., and Wing, R.R.
  1998   Reducing postpartum weight retention through a correspondence intervention. *In-
          ternational Journal of Obesity Related Metabolic Disorders* 22(11):1103–1109.
Nuckolls, K.B., Kaplan, B.H., and Cassel, J.
  1972   Psychosocial assets, life crisis and the prognosis of pregnancy. *American Journal of
          Epidemiology* 95(5):431–441.
Olafsdottir, A.S., Skuladottir, G.V., Thorsdottir, I., Hauksson, A., and Steingrimsdottir, L.
  2006   Maternal diet in early and late pregnancy in relation to weight gain. *International
          Journal of Obesity* 30(3):492–499.
Olson, C.M., and Strawderman, M.S.
  2003   Modifiable behavioral factors in a biopsychosocial model predict inadequate and
          excessive gestational weight gain. *Journal of the American Dietetic Association*
          103(1):48–54.
Olson, C.M., Strawderman, M.S., and Reed, R.G.
  2004   Efficacy of an intervention to prevent excessive gestational weight gain. *American
          Journal of Obstetrics and Gynecology* 191(2):530–536.
Orr, S.T., James, S.A., Miller, C.A., Barakat, B., Daikoku, N., Pupkin, M., Engstrom, K., and
Huggins, G.
  1996   Psychosocial stressors and low birthweight in an urban population. *American Jour-
          nal of Preventative Medicine* 12(6):459–466.
O'Toole, M.L., Sawicki, M.A., and Artal, R.
  2003   Structured diet and physical activity prevent postpartum weight retention. *Journal
          of Women's Health* 12(10):991–998.
Palmer, J.L., Jennings, G.E., and Massey, L.
  1985   Development of an assessment form: Attitude toward weight gain during preg-
          nancy. *Journal of the American Dietetic Association* 85(8):946–949.
Parker, B., McFarlane, J., and Soken, K.
  1994   Abuse during pregnancy: Effects on maternal complications and birth weight in
          adult and teenage women. *Obstetrics and Gynecology* 84(3):323–328.
Peterson, K.E., Sorensen, G., Pearson, M., Hebert, J.R., Gottleib, B.R., and McCormick,
M.C.
  2002   Design of an intervention addressing multiple levels of influence on dietary and
          activity patterns of low-income, postpartum women. *Health Education Research*
          17(5):531–540.
Picone, T.A., Allen, L.H., Schramm, M.M., and Olsen, P.N.
  1982   Pregnancy outcome in North American women. I. Effects of diet, cigarette smok-
          ing, and psychological stress on maternal weight gain. *American Journal of Clinical
          Nutrition* 36(6):1205–1213.
Polley, B.A., Wing, R.R., and Sims, C.J.
  2002   Randomized controlled trial to prevent excessive weight gain in pregnant women.
          International Journal of Obesity Related Metabolic Disorders 26(11):1494–1502.
Ricketts, S.A., Murray, E.K., and Schwalberg, R.
  2005   Reducing low birthweight by resolving risks: Results from Colorado's prenatal plus
          program. *American Journal of Public Health* 95(11):1952–1957.

Siega-Riz, A.M., and Hobel, C.J.
  1997 Predictors of poor maternal weight gain from baseline anthropometric, psychoso-
        cial, and demographic information in a Hispanic population. *Journal of the Ameri-
        can Dietetic Association* 97:1264–1268.
Stevens-Simon, C., and McAnarney, E.R.
  1992 Determinants of weight gain in pregnant adolescents. *Journal of the American
        Dietetic Association* 92(11):1348–1351.
  1993 Childhood victimization: Relationship to adolescent pregnancy outcome. *Child
        Abuse and Neglect* 18(7):569–575.
Stevens-Simon, C., Nakashima, I., and Andrews, D.
  1994 Weight gain attitudes among pregnancy adolescents. *Journal of Adolescent Health*
        14(5):369–372.
Walker, L.O.
  1995 Predictors of weight gain at 6 and 18 months after childbirth: A pilot study. *Jour-
        nal of Obstetric Gynecologic and Neonatal Nursing* 25(1):39–48.
  1997 Weight and weight-related distress after childbirth: Relationships to stress, social
        support, and depressive symptoms. *Journal of Holistic Nursing* 15(4):389–405.
Walker, L.O., and Freeland-Graves, J.
  1998 Lifestyle factors related to postpartum weight gain and body image in bottle- and
        breastfeeding women. *Journal of Obstetric Gynecologic and Neonatal Nursing*
        27(2):151–160.
Walker, L.O., and Grobe, S.J.
  1999 The construct of thriving in pregnancy and postpartum. *Nursing Science Quarterly*
        12(2):151–157.
Walker, L.O., and Kim, M.
  2003 Psychosocial thriving during late pregnancy: Relationship to ethnicity, gestational
        weight gain, and birth weight. *Journal of Obstetric Gynecologic and Neonatal
        Nursing* 31(3):263–274.
Walker, L.O., Freeland-Graves, J.H., Milani, T., Hanss-Nuss, H., George, G., Sterling, B.S.,
Kim, M., Timmerman, G.M., Wilkinson, S., Arheart, K.L., and Stuifbergen, A.
  2004 Weight and behavioral and psychosocial factors among ethnically diverse, low-
        income women after childbirth: I. Methods and context. *Women's Health* 40(2):1–
        17.
Wells, C.S., Schwalberg, R., Noonan, G., and Gabor, V.
  2006 Factors influencing inadequate and excessive weight gain in pregnancy: Colorado,
        2000–2002. *Maternal and Child Health Journal* 10(1):55–62.
Zimmer-Gembeck, M.J., and Helfand, M.
  1996 Low birthweight in a public prenatal care program. Behavioral and psychosocial
        risk factors and psychosocial intervention. *Social Science and Medicine* 43(2):187–
        197.
Zuckerman, B., Amaro, H., Bauchner, H., and Cabral H.
  1989 Depressive symptoms during pregnancy: Relationship to poor health behaviors.
        American Journal of Obstetrics and Gynecology 160(5 Part 1):1107–1111.

7

Emerging Themes

This report provides brief overviews of the workshop speakers' presentations and related deliberations and concludes with a set of emerging cross-cutting themes both for researchers interested in interdisciplinary work in this area and for those who are involved in developing strategies to promote appropriate weight before, during, and after pregnancy. The report should be viewed as only a first step in exploring opportunities to develop a synthesis of diverse research and applying this knowledge to promote appropriate weight in women of childbearing age, and it is confined to the material presented by the workshop speakers and participants. Neither the workshop nor this report is intended as a comprehensive review of what is known about maternal weight and gestational weight gain and maternal and child health outcomes, although it is a general reflection of the literature. Many additional contributors of gestational weight gain and health outcomes were not addressed in the limited time available for the workshop. A more comprehensive review and synthesis of relevant research knowledge will have to wait for further development.

Building from the initial presentations and deliberations, the committee has highlighted certain themes that are described below to help strengthen the direction and quality of future studies. One theme that arose early in the workshop was that the 1990 report of the Institute of Medicine (IOM), *Nutrition During Pregnancy*, was written at a time when concern was focused on insufficient gestational weight gain and concerns about low birth weight. In the intervening years, the larger context has shifted in light of increasing rates of obesity to create concern about too much weight gain during pregnancy and subsequent retention of weight, which may contribute to increasing obesity postpartum. The committee did not attempt to develop conclusions or recommendations in this activity. Given the wide range of methodological differences in the relevant research literature, a more extensive effort would be necessary to develop a critical review and analysis of evidence-based findings.

GESTATIONAL WEIGHT GAIN AND BIRTH WEIGHT

Gestational weight gain is an important variable of interest that has been studied extensively but deserves further attention. Gestational weight gain has three components: (1) the products of conception—that is, the fetus, the placenta, and the amniotic fluid; (2) the fluids in the extra tissue gained by the mother to support the pregnancy; and (3) maternal reserves. Roughly 70 percent consists of the pregnancy components and 30 percent is thought to be attributed to maternal stores. The largest component of gestational weight gain is water, followed by fat (the most variable of all of the components in the literature), and finally protein.

Patrick Catalano described the pattern of gestational weight gain, which is curved during the first two trimesters and then appears to be linear in the last trimester. Longitudinal studies of changes in fat mass show that as lean women (prepregnancy percentage of body fat of less than 25 percent) go through pregnancy, they tend to gain more fat compared with women who are obese (prepregnancy percentage body fat greater than 25 percent).

The IOM recommendations for weight gain in pregnancy reflect the curve of normal weight gain: very low at 0 to 10 weeks, 7 lbs. at 10 to 20 weeks, 10 lbs. at 20 to 30 weeks (this is when fat is accruing in the mother), and by 30 to 40 weeks the pace of weight gain should slow down. According to the average fetal growth curve, until about 28 weeks (the beginning of the third trimester), the average fetus weighs about 2 lbs. From 28 weeks until term, there is a 5.5 lbs. increase in weight that reflects fetal growth. Taken together, about 7.7 lbs. of weight in late pregnancy is related to the fetus, placenta, and amniotic fluid, not specifically maternal weight.

Past efforts to advise women on weight for pregnancy (before, during, and after) have focused little attention on maternal obesity. Most of the concern has addressed low birth weight deliveries in addition to other maternal and infant outcomes. However, a large increase in birth weight, concomitant with the increase in maternal weight over the last decade, is contributing to a shift in thinking about weight gain patterns and risks. It is important to note that measurement of birth weight is a proxy for several key indicators, including fetal growth and length of gestation. Low birth weight has additional causes other than gestational weight gain.

GUIDANCE FOR MATERNAL WEIGHT AND GESTATIONAL WEIGHT GAIN

The pregnancy weight recommendations of *Nutrition During Pregnancy*, the 1990 IOM report, were a frequent target of comment and discussion throughout the workshop. Other recommendations for pregnancy-related health were also noted, including guidance from the National Heart, Lung, and Blood Institute (NHLBI), the Maternal and Child Health Bureau, and the Centers for Disease Control and Prevention growth charts for adolescents. However, the prominence of the IOM recommendations in the work of the presenters and discussants was apparent. Of main concern were the need to reconcile different body mass index (BMI) categories (IOM versus NHLBI), the utility of and compliance with the IOM recommendations, and possible modifications to them.

BMI Categories

For different reasons, many speakers and discussants articulated the need to harmonize the BMI categories established by the IOM report, NHLBI, and others. The discrepancies were noted as challenges for both research (especially meta-analyses and cross-study comparisons) and clinical practice. The different BMI categories were also seen as a challenge to outreach efforts, as an apparent undermining of public confidence in the research and clinical community if apparently conflicting advice is disseminated.

Utility of and Compliance with IOM Recommendations

All speakers who presented data on weight gain patterns in reference to the IOM recommendations noted that only about one-third of women gained within the specified ranges during pregnancy; all others gained more or less weight than is recommended. It was not clear whether women reaching the recommended weight gain targets did so consciously or not, further raising questions about compliance (a similar point could also be made about missing the weight gain targets). Biologically, weight gain during pregnancy in a healthy woman is highly variable. A number of comments were made throughout the workshop about how to make the IOM recommendations more useful to women and to practitioners. Examples included further specification of special populations (obese, adolescents, other racial/ethnic groups) in terms of both target weight and BMI. Effective intervention methods are not understood.

The IOM Recommendations

Many comments were made about the need for further specification or modification of the existing IOM recommendations. The most commonly expressed view was that the recommendations needed to be updated, specifically for obese women and adolescents. This view was based on the history of the recommendations themselves, which were derived from research published before 1990 and did not consider the effect of weight gain on maternal outcomes of pregnancy. Given the sociodemographic changes seen in the population of pregnant women, many presenters indicated that revisiting the recommendations seems warranted. This effort should strive to link new recommendations directly to specific, and more diverse, pregnancy outcomes, especially since the incidence of low birth weight babies seems to be of less concern now than when the IOM recommendations emerged in 1990.

Several discussants also noted that more research is needed to investigate establishing recommendations (BMI cut-points) for pregnancy that reflect other health outcomes besides gestational weight gain and birth weight. For example, other maternal health outcomes could include postpartum weight retention, cardiovascular disease, and other metabolic issues; other child health outcomes could include obesity-related consequences (e.g., mental health, BMI, cardiovascular disease). There is a need to understand the risks and to maximize the benefits for mother and child.

Many related comments were definitional in nature—for example, clearly defining what components are included in gestational weight gain and determining when baseline weight should be taken (especially for multiparous women). There was also some discussion about adding gestational weight recommendations based on other indicators, such as abdominal girth, which are becoming strong predictors of negative outcomes.

SPECIAL POPULATIONS

The need to consider important subgroups within the general population emerged in several contexts. First, many studies show important interactions between predictor variables (socioeconomic status and education) and race/ethnicity, suggesting their importance generally but also underscoring implications for possible intervention efforts. When race/ethnicity is considered in the literature, major groups are underrepresented, including Asian, American Indian, and Hispanic groups. Similarly, the increasing rate of obesity has led to the emergence of a relatively new, and growing, group of women who are obese when they become pregnant. Finally, the discussion frequently led to consideration of adolescent pregnancy. Each of these is discussed below. Collectively, this theme centered on the need to provide more clarity, guidance, and interventions based on an individual's characteristics.

Diverse Racial/Ethnic Groups

Although researchers have become more likely to include racial/ethnic minorities in their studies, the effects by race and ethnicity are not always reported, and many studies do not conduct or report analyses looking for interaction effects with race and ethnicity. Across the studies reviewed in the course of the workshop, the influence of race and ethnicity is mixed, although certain relationships seems to emerge that could be more clearly communicated. For example, non-Hispanic black women retain more weight postpartum than white women in all BMI categories. Finally, research is emerging about cultural norms regarding pregnancy and weight that are not yet well understood.

Adolescent Mothers

Current consideration of pregnancy in adolescence and what guidance or interventions are appropriate for adolescent mothers with regard to obesity risk may need to be revisited. For example, the 1990 IOM recommendations suggest that very young adolescents gain up to the maximum of the range for their BMI. However, relative to older mothers, postpartum weight retention in young adolescents could be serious, as their lifetime weight retention risk may be far greater. For example, during the discussion, data presented about adolescent mothers suggested a relationship between adolescent growth during pregnancy and higher gestational weight gain and postpartum weight retention. In addition, many adolescent mothers (especially younger adolescents) would be expected to be gaining weight as part of typical development in the absence of a pregnancy. These biological factors, coupled with psychological and sociodemographic characteristics of adolescent mothers, make this a highly specialized population in need of focused attention.

Obese and Morbidly Obese Women

As obesity has increased generally, so has its incidence among women of childbearing age as well as among those who become pregnant. Obesity in women can cause serious pregnancy-related complications, but it can also be modified to improve birth outcomes. Additional attention is needed for the population of obese women who become pregnant. Several speakers suggested that prepregnancy BMI is a possible target for promoting appropriate weight during pregnancy and postpartum. Concerns were raised about reducing or controlling weight either before or during pregnancy through weight cycling, intentional weight losses, and regains. A number of practical issues also arise, especially for morbidly obese patients and those who were morbidly obese but underwent bariatric surgery or similar procedures before becoming pregnant. For example, medical practice and equipment may need to be modified to accommodate very large women during pregnancy and especially during delivery. Finally, obese women with a range of medical conditions in addition to their pregnancy can face additional challenges in the management of their pregnancy.

Lactating and Nonlactating Women

In general, breastfeeding is typically encouraged, if not supported, postpartum, for varying durations. However, lactation status is not a clear variable in research on gestational weight gain. Data are limited on potential mediating or moderating effects of lactation on maternal postpartum weight, as well as child outcomes.

THEORETICAL APPROACHES

Throughout the workshop discussion, participants offered a number of theoretical frameworks, either explicitly or implicitly. The workshop was not intended to bring about consensus on theoretical stance, but each of them suggested important considerations in promoting appropriate maternal weight and maternal and child outcomes.

Life-Course Approach

A number of speakers, discussants, and participants indicated that pregnancy is an event in the life course of the mother, yet few studies have integrated this approach into their designs. The clearest inclusion of the life-course consideration is in designs that incorporate parity. This has implications for research purposes as well as clinical practice. For example, data were presented showing the accumulation of weight following each birth, with the indication that weight gain in the first birth contributes to the prepregnancy weight in subsequent births, but the prepregnancy period for first-time mothers may be very different from that of mothers with children.

As discussed more fully in the context of interventions, the place and timing of a particular pregnancy in a woman's life also has implications for the types of interventions that may be necessary as well as those that may be feasible. Accounting for previous pregnancies is not the only consideration drawn from a life-course approach, however. A woman's age during pregnancy and childbirth has implications for her weight, gestational weight gain, health, and possibly child health outcomes. Delayed childbirth is driven by sociodemographic factors, which themselves could play a role, directly or indirectly, in maternal weight and health (cardiovascular disease) and child outcomes that are not necessarily explained by gestational weight gain.

Whole-Person Approach

Several participants drew on a whole-person approach, one that considers weight, nutrition, and physical activity as components of maternal weight status, gestational weight gain, and child outcomes. It was noted that the 1990 IOM recommendations address weight only. In general, nutrition for pregnant and lactating women is currently focused on caloric intake, without specific attention paid to specific nutritional requirements or guidelines. Calorie intake and good nutrition intersect when women make specific food choices. In addition to nutrition guidance, weight control is also about physical activity. It is also important to understand the biological variability in women. Individual metabolism affects calorie and physical activity outcomes. Studies indicate that the appropriate and inappropriate physical activity during and immediately following pregnancy is not well understood. It is important to understand different cultural traditions regarding food and physical activity during pregnancy when incorporating these variables in interventions to control weight.

The discussions noted that, in addition to food and physical activity, other psychosocial issues are important to examine in addressing the impact of pregnancy and its contributions to women's health. Although there are methodological problems in these studies of psychological factors, more research is needed.

Population and Individual Approaches

Several speakers noted the conflict between a population-wide approach and an individual approach, which focuses on specific cases. As with many areas of research and practice, this tension is exacerbated by large-scale studies that do not examine special populations or even individuals seen in a clinical setting. There is a need for guidelines, outreach, and education efforts driven by epidemiological research to be translated for practitioners treating individual women. In order to do this, more research is necessary to build a body of evidence about patterns in the general or selected populations that can be effectively communicated at the individual level.

INTERVENTION, OUTREACH, AND EDUCATION

Although one session of the workshop focused specifically on interventions or factors that affect appropriate weight during pregnancy and postpartum, the issues related to interventions came up repeatedly throughout the discussions. In general, few studies can be found in the literature that describe interventions for achieving appropriate weight before, during, and after pregnancy. Knowledge is therefore limited about appropriate study design, components, effective timing of interventions, and education and outreach. However, the discussion did produce some consistent themes that are highlighted below.

When to Intervene

A number of presenters and discussants commented on the importance of recognizing the timing of an intervention for achieving appropriate weight before, during, and after pregnancy. In some cases, this was driven by a general theoretical stance (i.e., the life-course approach discussed earlier) and in others it was driven by practical concerns. Advantages to intervening during the pregnancy were largely practical—a woman's visits to her medical provider are a great opportunity for an intervention. There is some regularity of contact between the woman and the medical provider, allowing for easier implementation of clinical-based interventions. However, many speakers noted concerns about balancing intervention goals with concerns about safety for the mother and the fetus during pregnancy, especially in connection with a restricted diet or heavy exercise. By contrast, interventions prior to or after pregnancy can focus on the woman without the same level of concern about the fetus, so more intensity may be possible. However, once women leave the prenatal treatment period, they are not regularly seen by the medical provider, making implementation a challenge. Several speakers noted high dropout rates in postpartum interventions although Special Supplemental Food Program for Women, Infants, and Children or regular infant care visits are possible points of contact postpartum. Nearly all who raised the issue, however, expressed an ideal that provided intervention before, during, and after pregnancy.

Components of Interventions

There is movement toward comprehensive interventions to promote recommended weight gain during pregnancy that focus on diet and physical activity, rather than a single-component approach. Psychosocial approaches are not well understood. In addition, designs using goal-setting with accompanying feedback to the woman were also noted to be essential components. Finally, although community-wide interventions were discussed and thought to be promising approaches, the very limited available research (one study) does not provide strong evidence for effectiveness.

Outreach and Education

Beyond specific interventions, attention was given to various outreach efforts to inform and educate women about weight, pregnancy, and health, addressed either to the medical community or to women in general as well as to pregnant or prepregnant women in particular. A number of speakers noted that pregnant women want information, yet they are reluctant to rely on information when it appears to be conflicting or ambiguous. The desire to provide useful information, for example, talking about nutritious food versus calories, was highlighted. A number of participants discussed how the media or a social marketing approach may or may not help in communicating information to women of childbearing age.

HEALTH CARE AND HEALTH SYSTEMS

Two themes arose during the discussion that concern health care and national health care systems. The first concerns the need for improved data collection systems to monitor maternal weight and weight gain during pregnancy and postpartum and report information on an epidemiological scale. The second focuses on practical implications of addressing maternal weight and weight gain during pregnancy and postpartum through health care systems in the United States.

Surveillance Systems

Currently no national surveillance system exists for monitoring weight and weight gain for pregnant women, nor for newborns and mothers postpartum, that would allow for tracking, documenting, and studying weight gain before, during, and after pregnancy. Although some states are attempting to use birth certificate data for these analyses, these efforts are still in the minority, and the data they collect are not standardized. To establish a surveillance system, however, critical decisions must be made about the data to be collected, the methodology, and the frequency. At various points during the workshop, participants indicated the need to collect data not only on height and weight (the necessary components for calculating BMI) but also on abdominal girth (although this latter measurement may be of little practical use when obtained during pregnancy). Measuring gestational weight gain at different time points throughout pregnancy is also seen as important in studying the effects of weight on child and maternal outcomes.

Once the data needs are identified, concerns about the validity of measurement must be considered, including local variability in definitions as well as variation introduced by differing data collection techniques, such as direct measurement versus self-report.

The Health Care System and Pregnant Women

The health care system for pregnant women is constrained by the nature and scope of services that are provided (or at least those that are accessible) to most women. For many first-time mothers, their entrance into prenatal care comes after conception and their health care providers provide relatively little education and information. Small changes to medical records could help professionals adequately track gestational weight gain. The lack of guidance from providers is especially likely for women who are uninsured or who have inadequate health insurance. This limited access to obstetric care is coupled with lack of access to other professionals, such as nutritionists and medical paraprofessionals, who could play an integral role in weight control programs and interventions. Health care disparities in the quality and cost of services for pregnant women are a wide-ranging problem. Pregnant women who typically show strong commitment to providing the best pregnancy they can for their unborn child simply lack access to intensive, multifaceted care. More systems-level studies are necessary, therefore, to strengthen the training of and access to quality care providers.

New mothers experience a transition with the birth of their child in their relationship with the health care system. Generally they have more regular access to pediatric care postpartum than maternal care. Applying a life-course approach to women before, during, and after pregnancy, there is need for alignment in the health care system across different care settings to ensure continuity of care for mothers with regard to their weight. A number of participants in the workshop noted that the current disconnected system (i.e., there is often no continuity of care for the woman before, during, and after pregnancy or with the care for the infant and older child) places limitations on collaborative efforts to control obesity.

SCOPE AND GAPS IDENTIFIED BY INDIVIDUALS DURING THE WORKSHOP

This list, which is based on the workshop discussions, reflects the suggestions made by presenters, discussants, and other workshop participants in relation to the workshop's task. It was prepared for the convenience of the reader. It should not be construed as representing recommendations or consensus statements.

1. Research and databases describing the distribution of maternal weight (prior to, during, and after pregnancy) among different populations of women (see Chapter 2).
    *   There is no national surveillance system that exists to adequately monitor maternal weight prior to, during, and after pregnancy in all racial/ethnic groups and different populations of women (e.g., adolescents and women of short stature) in the United States.
    *   No national representative data exist for some minority populations, including Asian, American Indian, Alaskan Native, and non-Mexican Hispanic women.
    *   Postpartum weight retention data are limited. Data show non-Hispanic black women retain more weight postpartum than non-Hispanic white women in all BMI categories.
2. Research and databases of the effects of different weight patterns (underweight and overweight) during pregnancy on maternal and child health outcomes (up to 12 months) (see Chapters 4 and 5).
    *   Data show an association of maternal prepregnancy BMI and a range of negative maternal and child health outcomes.
    *   Data show a relationship between gestational weight gain and negative maternal and child health outcomes.
    *   There are limited studies on the effects of pregnancy in adolescence.
3. Research available on the individual, community, and health care system factors that impede or foster compliance with recommended gestational weight guidelines (prior to, during, and after pregnancy) (see Chapters 3 and 6).
    *   The biological and social predictors or determinants reviewed may help women comply with recommended weight and gestational weight guidelines prior to, during, and after pregnancy.
    *   Data are limited on the individual, psychosocial, community-based, and health care and health care system factors reviewed that may help women comply with recommended weight and gestational weight guidelines during and after pregnancy. Data are especially limited on these factors and especially on the interactions of these factors.
4. Opportunities for Title V maternal and child health programs to help women of childbearing age to achieve and maintain recommended weight (prior to, during, and after pregnancy) (see Chapters 3 and 6).
    *   Data show prepregnancy BMI is a direct determinant of gestational weight gain. In addition, other research shows other biological and social determinants appear to influence the amount

(insufficient or excessive) and composition of gestational weight gain.

- Data are unclear about determinants of gestational weight gain among different populations of women.
- Studies are limited on interventions to promote appropriate weight during and after pregnancy.
- Presenters and discussants think a comprehensive intervention should be provided to promote recommended weight gain prior to, during, and after pregnancy rather than a single-component approach.

5. Future research and data collection efforts that could improve the efforts of Title V programs to support women from different racial and ethnic backgrounds in their efforts to comply with recommended weight guidelines and to improve their maternal health (see Chapters 2, 3, 4, 5, and 6).

- Collect representative data on the distribution of maternal weight (prior to, during, and after pregnancy) in all racial/ethnic groups in the United States.
- Additional research is needed to untangle the complex relationship of prepregnancy BMI (and other social and biological determinants) and gestational weight gain (rate and pattern of gain).
- Additional research is needed to understand the influence of biological and social determinants of gestational weight gain on different populations of women.
- Further research is needed on the effects of maternal weight and gestational weight gain (in combination and separate) on maternal and child health outcomes in all racial/ethnic and other populations of women (e.g., adolescents and women of short stature).
- Further research is needed on comprehensive (rather than single-component) interventions to promote recommended weight gain prior to, during, and after pregnancy.

FINAL OBSERVATIONS

Although this report was prepared by the committee, it does not represent findings or recommendations that can be attributed to the committee members. Indeed, the report summarizes views expressed by workshop participants, and the committee is responsible only for its overall quality and accuracy as a record of what transpired at the workshop. Presentations and discussion during the workshop on maternal weight gain during pregnancy highlighted a broad array of research topics, data elements, clinical interventions, and systems of care issues that are relevant to the influence of pregnancy weight on maternal and child health. Each of these areas revealed an evidentiary base that could contribute to in-depth analyses, but such studies are challenged by methodological limitations and gaps in the literature. Future efforts will need to draw on a variety of theoretical frameworks and special population studies as well as comprehensive epidemiological studies to shape clinical interventions and guidance for pregnant women in achieving healthy outcomes for all.

REFERENCE

Institute of Medicine
  1990   *Nutrition During Pregnancy.* Washington, DC: National Academy Press.

APPENDIX

Workshop Agenda
and Participants

WORKSHOP AGENDA

The Impact of Pregnancy Weight on Maternal and Child Health

May 30–31, 2006
National Academy of Sciences Building
Washington, DC

Tuesday, May 30

Welcome, Introduction, and Overview
Moderator: *Maxine Hayes, M.D., M.P.H.,* Committee Chair

8:30 am   **Welcome, Introductions, Background, and Overview of
Workshop**
Maxine Hayes, M.D., M.P.H., Committee Chair

8:45 am   **Overview: Trends in Maternal and Pregnancy Weight**
Mary Cogswell, R.N., Dr. P.H., Division of Nutrition
and Physical Activity, CDC
Patricia Dietz, Dr. P.H., Division of Reproductive
Health, CDC

**Panel 1: Gestational Weight Gain: Direct Predictors and Moderators and
Maternal Health Consequences**
Moderator: *Kathleen Rasmussen, Sc.D.,* Committee Member

9:25 am   **Biological and Metabolic Relationships**
Janet King, Ph.D., Children's Hospital Oakland
Research Institute

9:45 am   **Social Predictors or Relationships**
               Naomi Stotland, M.D., San Francisco, University of
               California

10:05 am   **BREAK**

10:20 am   **Short-Term Maternal Health Outcomes**
               Kathleen Rasmussen, Sc.D., Cornell University

10:40 am   **Long-Term Maternal Health Outcomes**
               Erica Gunderson, Ph.D., Division of Research, Kaiser
               Permanente Northern California

11:00 am   **Discussant Panel:**
               Each discussant will have 5 minutes.
                   Barbara Abrams, Dr. P.H., University of California,
                   Berkeley
                   Calvin Hobel, M.D., Cedars-Sinai Medical Center and
                   University of California, Los Angeles
                   Elizabeth McAnarney, M.D., University of Rochester,
                   Medical Center
                   Anna Marie Siega-Riz, Ph.D., University of North
                   Carolina, Chapel Hill

12:00 pm   **LUNCH**

**Panel 2: Maternal Weight and Gestational Weight Gain as Direct
Predictors and Moderators of Infant and Child Growth and Health**
Moderator: *Matthew Gillman, M.D.,* Committee Member

1:00 pm   **Short-Term Infant Health Outcomes**
               Patrick Catalano, M.D., MetroHealth Medical Center,
               Case Western Reserve University

1:20 pm   **Long-Term Child Health Outcomes**
               Emily Oken, M.D., Harvard Medical School, Harvard
               Pilgrim Health Care

1:40 pm   **Discussant Panel:**
                       Each discussant will have 5 minutes.
                          Mary Hediger, Ph.D., National Institute of Child Health and Human Development, National Institutes of Health
                          Michael Kramer, M.D., McGill University
                          Robert Whitaker, M.D., M.P.H., Mathematica Policy Research Institute, Inc.

2:40 pm   **BREAK**

Panel 3: Insights from Interventions to Promote Appropriate Weight During Pregnancy and Postpartum
Moderator: *Lillian Gelberg, M.D.,* Committee Member

3:00 pm   **Individual Approaches to Change Behaviors Related to Appropriate Weight During Pregnancy and Postpartum**
                          Rena Wing, Ph.D., Brown Medical School

3:20 pm   **Psychosocial-Related Factors That Affect Appropriate Weight During Pregnancy and Postpartum**
                          Lorraine Walker, Ph.D., University of Texas-Austin

3:40 pm   **Community Approaches to Promote Appropriate Weight During Pregnancy and Postpartum**
                          Christine Olson, Ph.D., R.D., Cornell University

4:00 pm   **Existing Practices and Policies for Clinicians and Health Systems Regarding Appropriate Weight During Pregnancy and Postpartum**
                          Laura Riley, M.D., Massachusetts General Hospital

4:20 pm   **Discussant Panel:**
                       Each discussant will have 5 minutes.
                          Edith Kieffer, Ph.D., University of Michigan, Ann Arbor
                          Carol Korenbrot, Ph.D., California Rural Indian Health Board
                          William McCarthy, Ph.D., University of California, Los Angeles

5:20 pm   End of the day

Wednesday, May 31

8:30 am **Continental Breakfast**

Summary of Previous Day

9:00 am *Moderator: Maxine Hayes (5–10 minute summary and then discussion)*
Review what is known about the distribution of maternal weight in different populations of women.

9:30 am *Moderators: Kathleen Rasmussen and Matthew Gillman (5–10 minute summary and then discussion)*
Review what is known about the effects of different weight patterns during pregnancy on maternal and child health outcomes.
• Based on the evidence presented, what else can be done to further improve maternal and child health outcomes?
• What research is needed to move the field forward?
• What have we missed?

10:15 am *Moderator: Lillian Gelberg (5–10 minute summary and then discussion)*
Review what we know about the individual, community, and health care system factors that (1) affect and (2) seek to improve maternal and child health outcomes through compliance with recommended gestational weight guidelines.
• To what extent are these policies and interventions based on scientific evidence presented around improving maternal and child health outcomes?
• Based on the evidence presented, what else can be done to further improve maternal and child health outcomes?
• Who needs to be involved to further improve maternal and child health outcomes? Is there a role for the media and public messaging?
• What research is needed to move the field forward?
• What have we missed?

12:00 pm End of Workshop

PARTICIPANTS

Barbara Abrams,* School of Public Health, Universisy of California, Berkeley

Tal Biron-Shental, Obstetrics and Gynecology, Washington University

Jeanne Blankenship, Western Human Nutrition Research Center, Agriculture Research Service, U.S. Department of Agriculture, University of California, Davis

Sarah Bonza, Department of Family Medicine, Ohio State University

Amy Branum, National Center for Health Statistics, Centers for Disease Control and Prevention, Hyattsville, MD

Jacquelyn Campbell, Institute of Medicine, The National Academies, Washington, DC

Amy Case, Birth Defects Epidemiology and Surveillance, Texas Department of State Health Services

Amanda Cash, Health Sciences Center, University of Oklahoma, Oklahoma City

Patrick M. Catalano, MetroHealth Medical Center, Cleveland, OH

Rosemary Chalk, Board on Children, Youth, and Families, National Research Council, The National Academies, Washington, DC

Diana Cheng, Women's Health, Maryland Department of Health and Mental Hygiene, Baltimore

Tae Chong, National Women, Infants, and Children Association, Washington, DC

Najmul Chowdhury, North Carolina Department of Health and Human Services, Raleigh

Cristina Churchill, National Research Center for Women and Families, Washington, DC

Mary E. Cogswell, Maternal and Child Health, Centers for Disease Control and Prevention, Atlanta, GA

Katsi Cook, Maternal and Child Health Coordinator, United South and Eastern Tribes, Inc., Tribal Epidemiology Center, Berkshire, NY

Ezra C. Davidson, Jr.,* Department of Obstetrics and Gynecology, Charles R. Drew University of Medicine and Science, Los Angeles, CA

Esa Davis, Family Medicine-Research Division, Case Western Reserve University, Cleveland, OH

Justine Desmarais, Women's Health, Association of Maternal and Child Health Programs, Washington, DC

Patricia M. Dietz, Division of Reproductive Health, Centers for Disease Control and Prevention, Atlanta, GA

Cathy Fagen, Long Beach Memorial Medical Center, CA

---

*Members of the program committee

Julie Farmer, Women, Infants, and Children, Omaha, NE

Robin Fleschler, University of Texas Medical Branch at Galveston

Frederic D. Frigoletto, Jr., Harvard Medical School, Boston, MA

Lillian Gelberg,* Department of Family Medicine, David Geffen School of Medicine, University of California, Los Angeles

Corrine Giannini, North Carolina Department of Health and Human Services, Raleigh

Matthew Gillman,* Department of Nutrition, Harvard Medical School and Harvard Pilgrim Health Care, Boston, MA

Gilman Grave, Endocrinology, Nutrition and Growth Branch, National Institute of Child Health and Human Development, National Institutes of Health, Department of Health and Human Services, Bethesda, MD

Nancy Green, March of Dimes, White Plains, NY

Erica P. Gunderson, Epidemiology and Prevention Section, Division of Research, Kaiser Permanente, Oakland, CA

Heidi Haddada, Office of Science and Technology, Washington, DC

Mary H. Hager, The American Dietetic Association, Washington, DC

Michelle Hansen, Colorado Department of Public Health, Denver

Maxine Hayes, (Chair),* State of Washington, Department of Health, Olympia

Mary L. Hediger, Epidemiology Branch, Division of Epidemiology, Statistics, and Prevention Research, National Institute of Child Health and Human Development, National Institutes of Health, Bethesda, MD

Calvin J. Hobel, Department of Obstetrics and Gynecology, Miriam Jacobs Chair in Maternal Fetal Medicine, David Geffen School of Medicine at University of California, Los Angeles

Mary Horlick, National Institute of Health, National Institute of Diabetes and Digestive and Kidney Diseases, Bethesda, MD

Kris Horning, Louis County Public Health, Lowville, NY

Edith C. Kieffer, School of Social Work, University of Michigan, Ann Arbor

Shin Kim, Centers for Disease Control and Prevention, Atlanta, GA

Janet King,* University of California, Berkeley and Davis, Children's Hospital Oakland Research Institute

Lisa King, Women's Health, Maternal and Child Health Bureau, Health Resources and Services Administration, Department of Health and Human Services, Rockville, MD

Sharon Kirmeyer, National Center for Health Statistics, Centers for Disease Control and Prevention, Hyattsville, MD

---

*Members of the program committee

Harriet Kitzman, School of Nursing, University of Rochester, NY

Luella Klein, Emory University, Gynecology and Obstetrics, Atlanta, GA

Ronald E. Kleinman,* Harvard University, Pediatric Gastroenterology, Boston, MA

Ann M. Koontz, Maternal and Child Health Bureau, Health Resources and Services Administration, Rockville, MD

Carol Korenbrot, California Rural Indian Health Board, Sacramento

Leslie Korenda, National Center for Health Statistics, Centers for Disease Control and Prevention, Hyattsville, MD

Michael S. Kramer, Pediatrics and Epidemiology and Biostatistics, McGill University, Quebec

Debra Krummel, University of Cincinnati, Nutritional Sciences, OH

Susan Landers, American Academy of Pediatrics, Austin, TX

Michele Lawler, Maternal and Child Health Bureau, Health Resources and Services Administration, Department of Health and Human Services, Rockville, MD

Stefanie Lee, Maternal, Child, and Adolescent Health, Office of Family Planning Branch, California Department of Health Services, Sacramento

Monique Lin, University of Alabama at Birmingham, Obstetrics and Gynecology

Jeanne Mahoney, American College of Obstetricians and Gynecologists, Department of Women's Health, Washington, DC

Sandra Mangum, Mississippi Department of Health, Jackson

Elizabeth McAnarney, Golisano Children's Hospital at Strong, University of Rochester Medical Center, NY

William McCarthy, University of California, Los Angeles, Johnson's Comprehensive Cancer Center

Chan McDermott, Texas Department of State Health Services, Austin

John McGrath, Information and Communication Branch, National Institute of Child Health and Human Development, Bethesda, MD

Elizabeth McGuire, Maternal and Child Health Bureau, Health Resources and Services Administration, Department of Health and Human Services, Rockville, MD

Michael Mennuti, American College of Obstetricians and Gynecologists, Department of Obstetrics and Gynecology, University of Pennsylvania, Philadelphia

Linda Meyers, Food and Nutrition Board, Institute of Medicine, The National Academies, Washington, DC

---

*Members of the program committee

Karen B. Mills, Capitol Area Human Services District, Nurse Family
Partnership Healthy Start, Baton Rouge, LA
Selina Mkandawire, Nutritionist (Private Practice), South Orange, NJ
Danielle Munro, Howard University Hospital-Women, Infants, and
Children, Washington, DC
Mandisa Nkrumah, Howard University Hospital Comprehensive Areas of
Resources, Entitlements and Services, Washington, DC
Emily Oken, Harvard Medical School, Harvard Pilgrim Health Care
Department of Ambulatory Care and Prevention, Boston, MA
Toni Olasewere, Mount Sinai Hospital, Obstetrics, Gynecology and
Reproductive Sciences, New York, NY
Christine M. Olson, Division of Nutritional Sciences, Cornell University,
Ithaca, NY
Therese Panagis, Arlington Department of Health Services/Public Health
Division, Family Health Services, VA
Gregg Pane,* Washington DC Department of Health
Estella Parrott, National Institute of Child Health and Human
Development, National Institutes of Health, Bethesda, MD
Kathleen Pellechia, Food and Nutrition Information Center, U.S.
Department of Agriculture, National Agricultural Library, Beltsville,
MD
Laura Peppelman, Delaware Women, Infants, and Children Program,
Dover
Terry Phan, Whitney Young Health Center, Albany, NY
Suzanne Phelan, Brown Medical School, Psychiatry and Behavioral
Medicine, Providence, RI
Maria Prince, Johns Hopkins Bloomberg School of Public Health,
Odenton, MD
Karlyn Probst, Virginia Healthy Start Initiative at Eastern Virginia
Medical School, Norfolk
Daniel Raiten, National Institute of Child Health and Human
Development, National Institutes of Health, Endocrinology,
Nutrition and Growth Branch, Bethesda, MD
Tonse Raju, National Institute of Child Health and Human Development,
National Institutes of Health, Bethesda, MD
Geetha Raman, Eastern Virginia Medical School, Norfolk
Leslie Randall, Northwest Portland Area Indian Health Board, Tribal
Epidemiology Center/CDC assignee, OR
Kathleen Rasmussen,* Division of Nutritional Sciences, Cornell
University

*Members of the program committee

Lauren Ratner, Association of State and Territorial Health Officials, Washington, DC
Eileen Resnick, Society for Women's Health Research, Scientific Programs, Washington, DC
Michael Rhone, Family and Consumer Sciences, Langston University, Oklahoma City, OK
Laura E. Riley, Vincent Obstetrics and Gynecology Service, Massachusetts General Hospital, Boston, MA
Sarah Roholt, Nutrition Services Branch, North Carolina Department of Health and Human Services, Division of Public Health, Raleigh
Vicki Lynn Rubio, Department of Human Services, State of California, Orange
Anne Santa-Donato, Associate Director, Childbearing and Newborn Programs, Association of Women's Health, Obstetric and Neonatal Nurses, Washington, DC
Jacquelyn Shufford, Crater Health District, Maternal and Child Health, Petersburg, VA
Anna Maria Siega-Riz, Department of Maternal and Child Health, School of Public Health, University of North Carolina, Chapel Hill
Janice Simmons, The Quality Letter for Healthcare Leaders, Alexandria, VA
Marcie Singleton, Knoxville County Health Department, Women, Infants, and Children Program, TN
Sharon Sirling, Maternal and Child Health Bureau, Department of Health, Honolulu, HI
Phillip Smith, Indian Health Service, Rockville, MD
Scott Snyder, Maternal and Child Health Bureau, Health Resources and Services Administration, Rockville, MD
Denise Sofka, Maternal and Child Health Bureau, Health Resources and Services Administration, Department of Health and Human Services, Rockville, MD
Leilani Spence, Health Department, Memphis and Shelby County Health Department, Memphis, TN
Catherine Spong, Pregnancy and Perinatology Branch, National Institute of Child Health and Human Development, Bethesda, MD
Julie Stagg, Texas Department of State Health Services, Family Health Research and Surveillance, Austin
Jamie Stang, University of Minnesota, Division of Epidemiology and Community Health, Minnetonka

*Members of the program committee

Susanne Strickland, National Institute of Child Health and Human Development, Office of Science Policy, Bethesda, MD

Naomi E. Stotland, Departments of Obstetrics, Gynecology, and Reproductive Sciences, University of California, San Francisco, San Francisco General Hospital

Laurie Tansman, Department of Clinical Nutrition, Mount Sinai Hospital, New York, NY

Judith Thierry, Indian Health Service, Office of Clinical and Preventive Services, Rockville, MD

Anjel Vahratian, University of Michigan, Obstetrics and Gynecology, Ann Arbor

Lorraine O. Walker, University of Texas at Austin, School of Nursing

Cindy Walton, Society for the Protection and Care of Children, Finger Lakes Women, Infants, and Children, Canadaigua, NY

Jennifer Weber, American Dietetic Association, Washington, DC

Gwendolyn West, Howard University Hospital, Washington, DC

Robert Whitaker, Mathematica Policy Research, Inc., Princeton, NJ

Rena Wing, Centers for Behavioral and Preventive Medicine, Weight Control and Diabetes Research Center, Miriam Hospital, Providence, RI

Allison Winter, Texas Department of State Health Services, Austin

Stella Yu, Research Branch, Maternal and Child Health Bureau, Health Resources and Services Administration, Department of Health and Human Services, Rockville, MD

---

*Members of the program committee